Also by Kathy Kaehler

Real World Fitness

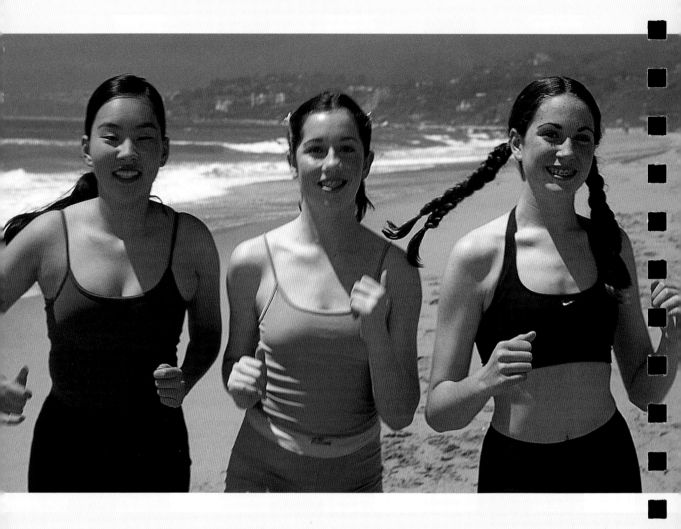

Cliff Street Books

An imprint of HarperCollinsPublishers

Teenage Fitness

Get Fit, Look Good, and Feel Great!

Kathy Kaehler

with Connie Church

HarperCollins books may be purchased for educational, business, or sales promotional uses. For information please write: Special Markets Department, HarperCollins Publishers, Inc., 10 East 53rd Street, New York, NY 10022.

FIRST EDITION

PRINTED IN CHINA

Designed by Celine Nadeau Vaccaro

Library of Congress Cataloging-in-Publication Data has been applied for.

ISBN 0-06-019863-X

01 02 03 04 05   IMX 10 9 8 7 6 5 4 3 2 1

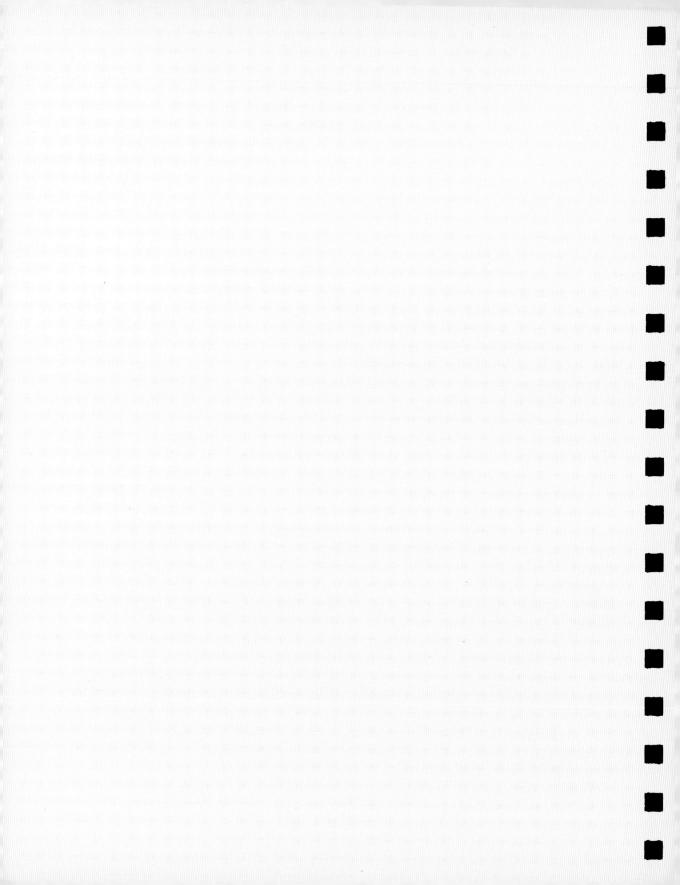

acknowledgments

Thank you to all of the girls who participated in this book. I hope that through your involvement other young women will be inspired to lead more natural, healthy, happier lives.

Eunice Kim	Andrea Mazey
Lauren Trainer	Taeler E. Cyrus
Gabrielle Miller	Melissa Hasbun
Lisa Grube	Eleanor Walker
Zoe Jackson	Marisa Walker
Alissa Bloch	Elaina Lombardo
Julia House	Alexi Wallace
Elizabeth Epps	Shannon Boyd

Dear Cooper, Payton, and Walker: I hope that someday you will read this book and understand the importance of maintaining a healthy body throughout your lives. Also, that you will influence others simply by setting a good example.

Acknowledgments

A special thanks to Kathleen Ingle for all your endless phone calls and running around. Kelly Auld, you were terrific for testing the five-minute workout. Thanks also to Nike for supplying the apparel and shoes; my photographer, Mike Russ, and his assistant, Danny Dougherty; Maria-Elena Arroy/Coutier for doing hair and makeup; and nutritionist Elizabeth Ward for your input.

—K.K.

A big hug and special thanks to my manager, Irene Webb of Infinity Management International. This is just our beginning!

To my three, beautiful, teenage girls whose angst about their bodies inspired me while working on this very necessary book.

And to my husband, Charlie, for being the best help he could be.

—C.C.

contents

chapter four   eating properly and breaking bad habits

chapter five

move it and use it

Introduction

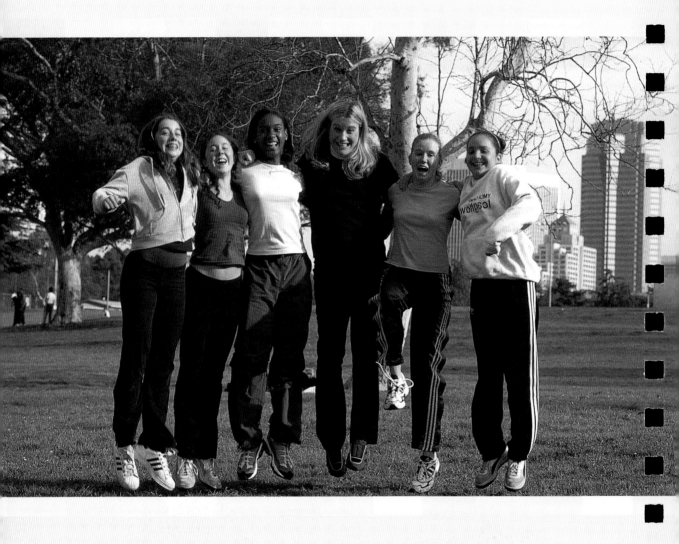

ou are a miracle, a gift from your parents. Since your life began, you've been nurtured and cared for, to become who you are today. As a teenager your care is not only the responsibility of those around you—but it begins to become yours. Eventually, no one else is going to take charge of your body.

The choices will be yours. On all levels, especially emotional and physical, your teen years are a period of tremendous transition. I like to think of this part of your life as a challenge. What better time, before you're completely on your own and while your body is naturally young and wholesome, to create a fitness plan that will allow you to lead a healthy, energetic, and meaningful life? I guarantee that when you are fit, you will have a greater ability to take control of your life and make decisions that are best for you. If you continue your fitness program into adulthood, you will be amazed at the abundant possibilities and opportunities that fill your life. You will also be surprised by the many challenges you are able to meet and overcome.

From the day I was born, I was a kid in perpetual motion. "Active" could have been my middle name. It's no wonder that gym class was my favorite and that I participated in every sport possible. My goal was to become a P.E. teacher. Instead, after college, my zest for fitness led me to numerous career opportunities, including aerobics director for Racquet World Health Club; one of the program directors at Jane Fonda's Laurel Springs Spa (wow!); my own training business (which still continues to grow), including celebrity clientele such as Drew Barrymore, Denise Richards, Claire Forlani, Cindy Crawford, Claudia Schiffer, and Michelle Pfeiffer; my first exercise video; my first book, *Real World Fitness*; and monthly magazine columns. To top it all off, for the last eight years I've been the fitness consultant on *Today*. That means the East Coast–West Coast trek on a regular basis.

Yep—all of this and a family too! Do I get tired? You bet I do, but all of the energy I put into my life just gives me the ability to do more!

This is not a "trendy" diet book or a magical fitness book. No, you will not wake up with thinner thighs in ten days. My goal is to help you develop a fit body *in a fun way* that you can expand on for the rest of your life. I want to share my energy and motivation with you so that you too will be able to eagerly take advantage of all the opportunities your life will bring.

I will teach you how to make your days more active without thinking you're exercising. Once you realize how good you feel and see the subtle changes that are beginning to happen to your body, you will see how being physically fit is easy and anyone can achieve it. I have provided two workouts that you can do regardless of where you are.

Exercise alone will not work. Nutrition plays an essential role as well. I will thoroughly discuss healthy food guidelines and easy-to-follow eating habits, though I'm not going to provide you with a specific diet to lose weight. It won't work because you're growing and changing every day. All that is required for you to reach a healthy weight for your height and bone structure is to eat from the different food groups in a balanced and moderate way. And activity is required. Lots of physical activity.

This is what fitness is all about. It's that fine balance between the right amount of physical activity and proper nutrition. Fitness is not about having a perfect body—an impossible and highly subjective goal anyway. Fitness is about having a body that feels good!

Ideally, this book will get you started on a fitness path that you can follow for the rest of your life. You can't imagine what some adults go through who have put it off. They believed how they looked in their teens and twenties would last forever. Suddenly different parts of their bodies sagged, they found themselves winded after going up one flight of stairs, and they might be dealing with health problems that originate from a lack of activity. Not knowing what to do, they try every crazy diet under the sun and spend tons of money on workout equipment they rarely use. And they have no concept of the words *moderation* and *consistency*.

This book will provide you with the best tools for integrating fitness into your life. And believe me, good fitness habits practiced now will eventually become as automatic as brushing your teeth. Once established, it's a routine you'll never stop.

Since fitness has been a part of my life for as long as I can remember, I made a lot of good choices early on that help me with my body, help me have a successful career, and help me manage my life today. But it wasn't always this way.

When I was younger, because I didn't think I looked perfect

enough, I made many bad choices involving my diet that taught me some hard lessons. Due to my bad body image, I had to get seriously ill first with bulimia before I could begin to get genuinely fit. I even ended up hospitalized a couple of times—talk about humiliating and embarrassing! The first thing I want to do is share my personal story with you so maybe, just maybe, I can help you avoid those bad, at times fatal, fitness habits.

When you finish this book, I hope you realize that this is the optimal time in your life to take control of your body by taking action, carefully choosing your food and exercise options, as your future is taking shape. Regardless of body basics that you can't change, such as your height and bone structure, one opportunity everyone has is to become physically fit! With physical fitness come mental stamina, confidence, an external glow, and an inner strength that nobody can take away from you—it lights that internal flame, the motivation to do everything better.

Never forget that your body is a miracle and that you are the one who is in charge of it. And appreciate—appreciate everything that makes you unique from the top of your head to the tip of your toes!

chapter one

Kathy's Story

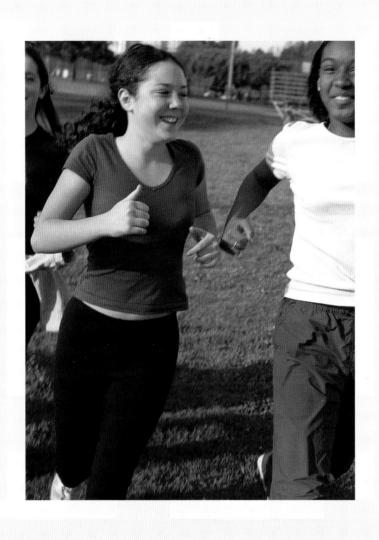

on the road again!

my family did a lot of moving around during my elementary and high school years. We moved to São Paulo, Brazil, when I was five years old and came back to the States when I was eleven. I went to school in Michigan until I was in the ninth grade, and moved to Wisconsin for tenth grade. During my eleventh- and twelfth-grade years, I was back in Michigan.

All this change was a huge challenge for me. It was hard leaving old friends behind and then having to make new friends wherever and whenever we moved. What saved me, time and time again, was my love for sports. I was always on a team, so I always made friends very quickly.

Even in kindergarten I was competitive. I would beat all the boys in my gym class and continued to do so through junior high school. I couldn't wait for gym class, because my gym teachers would always use me to demonstrate the day's physical challenges.

my role model

From sixth through eighth grade, I had the best gym teacher, Miss Reider. What a great role model for a young teen! She was very feminine and yet very athletic; she drove a blue Camaro and had a glorious mane of long blond hair. I idolized her. So, of course, gym was my favorite class.

Presidential physical fitness awards were a big part of my life. It was simply a given that I had to be in the top percentile. I was competing with myself, my classmates, and the whole school for ranking. This was something that really mattered, and it made me dig deep within myself to win. All the other teachers in the school knew who was performing at the top, so it made me feel that everyone cared.

the all-american "cute"

At this point in my life, I don't remember thinking about the shape of my body. I was so active all the time that I never thought about perfection or if I was thin enough. My body was the way it was, and that was that! And constant activity kept it the way I wanted it.

In high school, I made the first string in several sports, including cross-country running, volleyball, basketball, and the track team. I was also heavily involved in the drama and music departments. How did I do so much? I had so much energy from being physically fit.

The stress and pressure of being thin didn't start until the eleventh grade. I was popular, but I didn't have a boyfriend like the other popular girls. I think this was the beginning of what led to the eating problems I developed later.

In the twelfth grade, everything finally came together. I played all sports and ran in events that took me to the state championships. I sang in the choir and got the lead role in the musical *Hello, Dolly!* I excelled in my studies, got a boyfriend, and surprisingly found myself on the homecoming court. I was finally seen as the all-American girl, athletic and cute.

my obsession with *thin* begins

I should have been feeling pretty good about myself, but the feelings of *"not thin enough"* started to haunt me. They came out of nowhere. Suddenly my appearance became everything. I was obsessed. To whom was I comparing myself? Other girls in my class? And did I think being thinner would somehow change things?

I had to leave for school at 7:00 A.M. I got up extra early to do the full "prep" before I left: shower, hair, makeup, perfect outfit, and I packed up all the little necessities I was going to need throughout the day to maintain my appearance.

how not to eat

Mom insisted that I couldn't leave the house without eating breakfast. Fortunately for me, she was busy in and out of the kitchen, so I could "fake" my breakfast. I would crumble up little bits of toast in my bowl, pour some milk over the crumbs, and swish it around so that it looked like I was eating. If I had eaten, those measly calories would have been easily burned off by 10:00 A.M.

At about this time, I started going to the drugstore and buying over-the-counter diet pills (which later in life almost killed me). These diet pills took away my appetite and made me feel very jittery.

When I look back at pictures of me at that time of my life, I have no idea why I was taking a diet pill. My dysfunctional eating and dieting never got too out of hand at this point, but my insecurity with guys intensified when my boyfriend dumped me with a note (coward!) and started seeing a girl who ran on my relay team. He was a jerk, and I was crushed. Even though all of this had happened, I still managed to have a memorable senior year.

phys. ed.

College meant another new school and making new friends. I was accepted at Hope College in Michigan, a mere four hours away from home.

As a physical education major, I was in the athletic department nonstop. Once again on the volleyball team, with a shot to be on varsity. This was great, and I felt very at home, but the old insecurities surfaced. To make matters worse, I was slowly gaining weight.

phys. dead!

Partying" was something new to me. I hardly drank alcohol in high school, but college was a different story.

I met a girl in the dorm who showed me a magical trick involving your finger. After partying and bingeing, she took me down to one of the basement bathrooms and stuck her finger far back in her throat to make herself vomit. Then she went to bed feeling guiltless about what she'd consumed because she'd gotten rid of it all—or so she thought.

At first I struggled with it. And it was gross! But everything she'd eaten was gone when she did it. So I stuck with it and voila! It was my green light to eat without worrying. What I didn't know was that bingeing and purging isn't a very good way to lose weight. Why? Because you are ingesting way too many calories when you binge, so you may remain at the same weight. This is what was happening to me.

out of control

I started taking diet pills again. I would eat anything in private and then feel like killing myself until I found a toilet and threw up. Ah—I thought I was back in control. Then I would swallow a diet pill, and I'd be stimulated until I was really hungry and desperate to eat again, because I had gotten used to eating huge amounts of food. So I'd binge again and then purge again. I was completely out of control. I had become a diet pill–popping bulimic!

I don't know at exactly what point this happened, but I'd been on the vicious binge-purge-pill cycle for a while, and I had increased the number of diet pills I was taking. These were the very potent kind loaded with extra caffeine. I was on my way out of the dorm when everything suddenly started spinning and then went black.

The next thing I remember was the paramedic kneeling next to me, asking me where I was from and what month it was. I didn't know the answers. Later at the hospital, when I was more coherent, I was told that I'd had a seizure. The doctors wanted to know all about my medical background and lifestyle.

When you're bulimic, you learn to lie quite well. I had been lying to my friends, my family, and anyone else who crossed my path. I was released from the hospital without revealing anything except that I was lacking sleep.

in
over my head

Another year passed and—oh man—was I in deep. I was throwing up everything I ate. Food was the "devil" to me when it was inside me. Right before and during the binge-purge cycle I was out of control. Then I'd take the diet pills, swearing I was giving my old habits up for good. I was like an alcoholic on a roll, swearing he was taking his last drink! Who was I kidding?

One day I had binged, thrown up, and swallowed five extra-strength diet pills. I was on my way to a friend's place off campus. I remember everything starting to spin, as before, and then I blacked out. Somehow I made it across the street without being hit by a car, went into a market, bought a soda, and then had my second *grand mal* seizure.

Once again, I woke up to a paramedic at my side. As he stood over me, he asked who the president of our country was. I was clueless. At the hospital, I knew what my problem was. An intern, a big, healthy-looking woman, was fussing over me and I started talking to her. I asked her if a seizure could be caused by some of the stuff I had been doing. She emphatically answered yes and told me that the next time could be my last time.

I could die from the crazy stuff I was doing to my body! And all for the sake of *thin*.

The big, healthy intern had told me so. Without a doubt, my lifestyle was killing me. And it had to change.

scared straight

These seizures scared me straight. I had to learn how to eat right, sleep enough, and get the right amount of exercise. Don't be misled—it was tough.

I would have conversations with myself about how if I ate too much, I would be tempted to throw up. I talked myself into keeping it down. Attached to the amount I ate was the constant thought of having a seizure at home with my parents watching and how scared they would be seeing me have one. With all this fear racing around inside me, I was able to change my mind-set and talk myself out of bingeing throughout the summer, as I took it one day at a time. I congratulated myself at the end of each day.

I never intentionally threw up again. In fact, to this day, it really bothers me if I happen to get food poisoning or the flu and have to throw up.

truly fit at last

After my college graduation, I was extremely fortunate to land an internship at the Coors Wellness Center in Golden, Colorado. The center was at the Coors Beer Company, which had started the first corporate fitness program in the country.

They had three interns a year who would have the opportunity to work with one of the staff members there. Once I moved to Colorado, I realized the important role health and fitness played in the residents' lives. It was great to see everyone looking so healthy and fit.

Every day I found myself in situations where I was around people whom I emulated as I learned how to eat and exercise properly. I began to understand how the body works to utilize food and maintain lean muscle mass.

I helped people who didn't have much activity or exercise in their lives by creating programs that worked with their desires and constraints. I'd watch them blossom as a result of my coaching and training. I found that I was good at helping people develop their determination to change. I got them to the point where exercise felt as natural and regular to them as getting dressed for the day.

I had some brief bouts of fighting off my old eating disorder, but I was continuing to recover without any slips. What better environment for me to be in? I gave talks to the people in the program about eating disorders and told my story. I was surprised at what I learned about myself. And I discovered that a great number of others suffered from eating disorders as well.

working in the real world!

After completing my internship, I stayed in Colorado and took a job at a health club in Denver. This club had hired many of the interns from Coors. The director of the club's wellness center, Dr. Daniel Kosich, hired me to work on a special weight-loss program he had created called Fatburners. The program involved one-on-one training, a nonimpact aerobics class, and educational lectures. There was also pre- and post-program testing that included body fat testing, a treadmill stress test, blood pressure and cholesterol screening, and a custom exercise program design. The people who participated in this program claimed it changed their lives. It also changed mine. I knew that working one-on-one with people was what I wanted to do.

my first taste of celebrity

I had learned so much from Dr. Kosich that I was sad yet so excited for him when I learned he was leaving for California to work with Jane Fonda. He would be her new consultant for all the videos, books, and products ahead and classes for which she was already so famous. Jane was starting a new spa. When she came to him for advice on whom he thought should work there, he thought of me. I couldn't believe my good fortune when I heard that I was being considered for this job!

I had to fly to Santa Barbara—a small, coastal, vacation city not far from Los Angeles. Dr. Kosich met me at the airport, and we drove up to the spa.

I'll never forget the long, curvy road we traveled on until we pulled up before a huge gate. Laurel Springs was a country farm estate, with barns for the animals and lodge-style buildings. As I got out of the car, at a little cottage, I looked up and saw Jane Fonda, with that beautiful smile, striding across the lawn to greet us. My palms were sweaty as I shook hands with the first famous person I'd ever met.

Jane's presence is awesome. She took my breath away that first day. I haven't felt the same intensity since—not even when I met Barbra Streisand, Michelle Pfeiffer, Arnold Schwarzenegger, and other celebrities in the course of my fitness-training career.

My interview with Jane began with a grueling hike, and she really kicked my butt as she paced herself ahead of me all the way! She was fifty, and I was a very physically fit woman in her mid-twenties. I tried to conceal my huffing and puffing!

Next, I was to teach her a one-on-one aerobics class. It took all the courage and brains I could muster to teach the "queen of aerobics" unique variations of what I knew. Afterward, I was pooped, but Jane headed for the pool to swim a few laps.

We finished up in the gym, discussing my lifelong experience with fitness. Then she explained to me that Laurel Springs was a spa designed for one-on-one personal training. Many of the clients were in the entertainment business and were veterans of trendy diets, exercise fads, and other obsessions related to food and working out. Jane wanted someone to join the staff who could bring some honesty and realism to the spa, someone who could teach her clients how to change their lives through healthy eating habits and exercise. She was looking for consistency and simplicity in the approach.

Jane shared some of her personal experiences with me, and it turned out that we'd had similar problems in the past with dieting. As the interview ended, I felt that we really had hit it off and that I could provide her clients with what they needed. Fitness didn't need to be complicated to work.

The next day I was called and told I had the job. This brought me into the celebrity realm and changed my life forever. During the year I worked at Laurel Springs, I trained one-on-one with a number of Jane's friends, including Rue McClanahan, Sharon Gless, Melanie Griffith, and Ally Sheedy.

When the Laurel Springs Spa closed, I took my career a step further and started contacting the celebrities I had trained. Many were eager to continue working with me, so I started my own personal-training business. By 1990, I was building a solid career helping people get fit and feel good about themselves. Financially, I was self-supporting, doing what I loved. Things couldn't have been better.

oops! i did it again!

It happened again. I don't know why; maybe it was because of all the celebrities and how great they appeared, but the old feelings started to come back about how I looked. It made no sense. I was teaching aerobics three times a night and my body looked great. Still, the insecurity about my looks lingered and my wanting to get thinner took hold of me and made me resume a crazy, unhealthy lifestyle.

I was driven. I was motivated to get more clients, whatever the cost. Needless to say, I was not paying attention to my own physical needs, but there was no bingeing and purging. I kept my promise.

This time it was virtual starvation all day while training my clients—except for several coffees throughout the day and my morning apple fritter—and then often I'd go out all night. Sometimes I'd have wine, a small meal, and maybe some more wine. I was spending my nights with a very famous actor who liked to live on "the edge." He said he loved my body, not knowing it was a body that was about to self-destruct.

Once again, I was putting my life in jeopardy. I was living on no sleep, the endorphins from my aerobics classes, the stimulation from the caffeine in the coffee, and the excitement of this very steamy relationship.

I thought I'd never have another seizure, because I wasn't throwing up. But I did. And it occurred while I was on a hike with a client. My client was so worried about me, but I was embarrassed and ashamed. I knew why it had happened.

acceptance and forgiveness

This time it was over. I faced myself honestly: Kathy Kaehler was killing herself. Kathy Kaehler was finally convinced that she had to change her lifestyle for good.

I had to turn it around.

I had to turn around and focus on getting healthy—and fast! This was not to be a Band-Aid cure. This was a for-the-rest-of-my-life change. And it would have to include some mental and spiritual adjustments as well. My gut told me there would be no more chances. What a hypocrite I had been! Teaching fitness to others while not practicing the basic principles myself.

I chose to accept the strong, healthy body I was born with (far from perfect—whatever that really is) and appreciate its uniqueness and all that it could do. My body was a miracle, and here I'd been taking it for granted. I forgave myself for all the abuse I'd put it through. It was important that I released any guilt I felt. I knew I could always start again. (Any of us can!) Move on and look at all the opportunities I'd have to pursue in my life as I anticipated my future.

As this reality finally sank in, another realization came with it and has stayed with me. I learned that it didn't matter what other people thought of me, as long as I felt good about myself and was doing what I loved to do while accomplishing my goals. I was able to immerse myself in my work completely and to stop worrying about when I was going to meet someone special. I felt a sense of relief as I accepted the fact that I am the only one who is going to look out for me.

The Cinderella story is more than a fairy tale—it's a setup. There are no knights in shining armor coming to save me—or any of us. I am the knight on the horse who must direct the course my life will take. It's up to me to make choices and take the appropriate actions.

Shortly after this revelation, I met my wonderful husband of seven years. I love being married to Billy and raising our three boys, but I still consider myself responsible for me. And I always will.

chapter two

Mirror, Mirror on the Wall

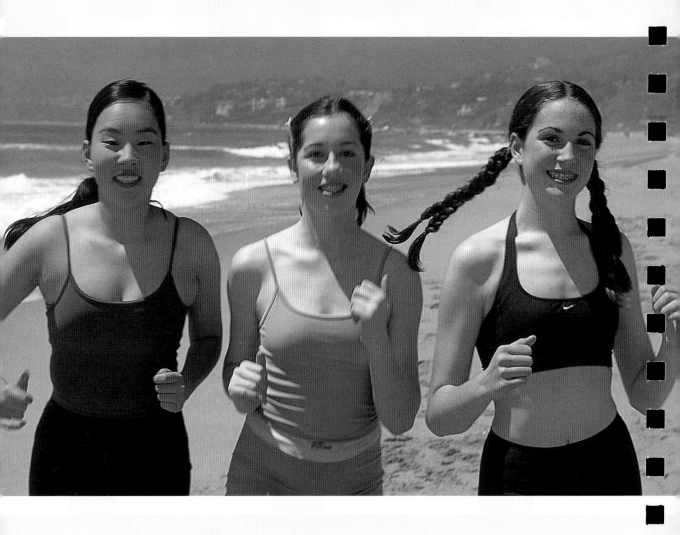

the teenage girl's rite of passage

your teen years should be the most exciting, vivacious years of your life! Of course your schoolwork is important, but this time is also filled with movies, concerts, the phone, fashion consciousness, collecting girlfriends, and sharing secrets. Also, there are the two big D's to look forward to, dating and driving, and all of the special events that are a part of both: football games, homecoming, dances, proms, parties, that first "special" guy, maybe your first car (for better or worse), and your first real summer job.

During this rite of passage to "periods," "pubes," "boobs," and "dudes," it's normal to feel physically and emotionally awkward and out of sync at times. Believe me, you're not alone, as every teen is right there with you—this includes the guys too! So lighten up. It's okay to let yourself act silly, carefree, and a bit outrageous as long as you balance it all with a daily routine that includes enough sleep, wholesome, yummy food, and exercise.

Fortunately, I found many teens' points of view about this "rite of passage" refreshing. Some of the girls I interviewed told me:

"I love sports because they're so much fun. And I think 'fun' is prettier than the perfect makeup because it's real. Of course I know how to play up my physical assets when I'm going to a party or out on a date. And that's fun too."

—*Shannon, age 16*

"I don't weigh myself and only spend fifteen minutes getting ready for school! If you're a strong enough person, you can get past all the social pressure of how you should look. I like to think my good habits are a part of keeping me fit."

—*Zoe, age 17*

"I'm glad people are drawn to my big, blue eyes. I'll never forget the glamour of my first homecoming—but I'm about a lot more than the makeup and the slinky dress. I make sure I work out at least four days a week and munch on veggies and fruit when I study!"

—*Elaina, age 16*

"My first kiss felt so strange. Neither one of us knew what we were doing. I bet I turned eight shades of red. I'm just thankful the front porch light was out."

—*Lindsey, age 15*

"Well, my body is far from perfect and I definitely have to improve my fitness level. But I have so many friends because I am a good friend. And I could spend hours on the phone. I don't think being a freshman in a big high school is so bad, even though there are so many gorgeous, skinny girls all over the place."

—*Marisa, age 14*

The flip side to all of the fun, jeopardizing any girl's self-esteem, is the pressure she can feel every time she looks into the mirror during this period of her life. Trying to live up to impossible expectations, she believes she is: *not pretty enough, not thin enough, not popular enough*. These beliefs can develop into more than a bad attitude.

From the increase in drinking, drugs, depression, and eating disorders to a higher suicide rate—all of it makes me realize how terrifying the world has become for our kids. Teens are so focused on their physical and emotional selves that they seem to have forgotten about their intellect, spirituality, and having harmless fun, whatever forms these may take. It seems that regardless of the quality of their upbringing, they place a dramatic emphasis on the superficial aspects of their lives. Consequently, they will go to any lengths to get the look and attention they want. Before they know it, they're teetering on the brink of self-destruction. Here comes the balance theory again. When there is no balance, eventually something, if not everything, is going to give. Remember my story? It's the perfect example of what happens to your mind, body, and spirit when you either live on very little food (and bad food at that) or binge and purge, put in long hours of hard work, obsess over a guy, get very little sleep, and have too much physical activity.

I'm sad to say that for every positive point of view there was also a negative one. Other girls I interviewed told me:

"Even though I wear a size three, if I was a thinner person I know I would be happy. Since I'm not, I do stupid things to my body like shave my eyebrows to redesign my eyes and change my hair color every two weeks even though it's starting to fall out. I've also eaten a whole bag of potato chips and then made myself puke because I was afraid my waistline would turn into a balloon."

—*Alexi, age 14*

"Being thinner means I'll start liking my body and wear the two-piece bathing suit my mom bought me. I wish I didn't care how I look in it, because we shopped together to find just the right one to make me feel less self-conscious while I lose weight. Mom was very patient and spent a lot of money. I haven't had the courage to wear it yet, and the summer is almost over!"

—*Ellen, age 15*

"I started getting too thin because I got mononucleosis and lost my appetite. After I was well, I decided I liked my 'new skinny look' because it made me prettier—like a fashion model. Then it became fun to see how thin I could continue to get. My doctor said I was on the verge of being anorexic."

—*Eleanor, age 16*

"I never want to wear a size ten like my cousin does. She's my age and she just seems so big. Sure, she's a few inches taller—but size ten sounds like a tent size to me. So I live on low-cal shakes, dry toast, and lots of vegetables. Dinner? Most of it ends up in my napkin and then in the garbage. And I run at least three miles every day!"

—*Linda, age 15*

the type of the "hype"

Today's role models certainly aren't helping teens get fit. Helping teens get fit is a cause that I consider my personal mission. Most actresses, and of course models, feel that they must be SKINNY in their fight to remain competitive in an industry where "thin is always in." As

you page through a magazine and see a beautiful, lean model, you probably think that you'd give anything to be built like her. But at what price?
By starving yourself? By bingeing and purging like I did?

What is anorexia nervosa? This is a relentless pursuit of
thinness that leads to the refusal to eat and can result in
extreme loss of weight, hormonal disturbances, and death.
Symptoms include:

- refusal to maintain normal body weight for height and
  age
- weighs 85 percent or less than what is expected for age
  and height
- menstrual periods stop or do not begin at the appropriate age
- person is terrified of becoming fat, or gaining weight
  even though she is seriously underweight
- complains of feeling fat although she's very thin
- also, an anorexic will be depressed, irritable, and with-
  drawn

What is bulimia nervosa? This is binge eating that is followed by self-induced vomiting. Symptoms include:

- person binge eats excessively
- feels out of control while eating
- vomits, uses laxatives, exercises, or fasts to get rid of the calories
- starts a new diet when not bingeing, but eventually starts the bingeing cycle again
- places total self-worth in being thin
- often shoplifts, is promiscuous, and abuses alcohol and drugs
- person's weight may be normal or near normal—unless anorexia is present as well
- bulimics may put up a cheerful front, while secretly they feel lonely, depressed, and ashamed inside

Many teens practice either one, or both, not realizing the devastating health consequences being inflicted on their bodies. They may also try other extreme diets combined with intense exercise programs, to conform to strong social pressures that declare thin as popular.

Thin doesn't always mean fit! Without having flexibility, strength, and cardiovascular fitness, fashion models are not fit—unless they're bionic! Who knows what's really going on with their bodies? If they're thin because they're eating balanced meals and exercising, or were born with that body type (Cindy Crawford is a good example) and have a high metabolism—great! They're lucky! But if they're thin because of eating disorders, a misuse of laxatives, and/or are using drugs, then it's all an illusion. And you're buying into it.

I worry about teens caught up in the thin industry. They may not be "clinically anorexic," but their bony, unnatural frames and rail-thin, dangling arms lead me to believe that many don't have healthy eating habits. Add to this long school days, maybe an after-school job, arduous physical workouts, and little sleep, and you've got unhealthy daily routines.

Thank God I, one of the most naturally healthy people I know, finally came to my senses and started getting truly physically fit before I accidentally killed myself. With every bit of self-discipline I had, I took control of my eating habits, finally properly fueling my very active body on a consistent basis.

Many celebrities look to me to help them get physically fit. I have to constantly remind them that besides their workout program, they have to eat well-balanced meals daily. For many it's a struggle because they are convinced that food is the "devil" and will somehow undermine their chances of success. Believe me, as gorgeous as you think they are, they have their insecurities about their bodies. Some are terrified of not getting a part or getting bumped from a show if they don't look good enough. They fear not looking perfect in that designer gown made just for them for a special awards show. And of course there's the age factor. I have a huge responsibility in helping these people. The fact that so many people put their bodies in my care is very flattering.

I know you'd like to look like some of the people I work with and train. I get letters from many of you, and my favorite standard question is "What can I do to have arms like Denise Richards?" My response now is, "Well, you'll have to call up her manager and see if you can have some type of surgery that will remove her arms and attach them to yours! In truth, you have your own arms, and you can't have somebody else's."

The good news is that there are lots of exercises to improve your body's appearance. But before you begin to work on your body, you must change your mind-set from the "I want to look like her" way of thinking. It does nothing for you but lead to frustration, despair, and low self-esteem. The only solution is to accept yourself as you are, and then get busy making yourself physically fit. Focus on your assets!

you can change your mind-set

One way to turn your mind-set around is by incorporating the following three words into your fitness vocabulary each day. You might want to spend five minutes a day meditating on these words and what they truly mean to you in a positive way. They are: *acceptance, change,* and *consistency*.

acceptance: believing in what God gave you. This means working with what you've got—not with what you don't have.

change: working with what you have. This means enhancing the best of what you've got by balancing exercise and physical activity with your food intake.

consistency: in your approach to eating and exercise. With this comes the word *sensible*.

understanding your body type or somatype

Hilary Swank could play her Oscar award–winning part in *Boys Don't Cry* because of her *natural* body type. She has a boyish figure with straight up-and-down legs. No curves. Exercise and diet did not give Hilary Swank her body—it's in the genes.

Teens seem to crave this boyish look. I always tell them, quite frankly, "Well, if you'd like to turn in your vagina and uterus for a penis—then you'll be able to go without those upper thighs and hips. Though, you might wish you had them during your pregnancy!"

Yes, there are some girls whose hips and thighs are stick-straight because, like Hilary Swank, it's their body type. But I always tell a teen who is hung up on her hips and thighs to think ahead: women are meant to carry babies and to give birth. That's why they have wider hips than men.

One of the best things you can do for yourself is learn what your body type or somatype is and accept it. This should remove a lot of the pressure you're apt to put on yourself to look perfect.

The three genetic somatypes are: *ectomorphs, mesomorphs,* and *endomorphs*. Most of you will primarily relate to one of these types, but many of you have supportive traits from a second type.

If you are an ectomorph, you naturally have a small bone structure, low body fat, a small amount of muscle mass and muscle size, and a high metabolism.

As a mesomorph you naturally have a medium to large bone size, low to medium body fat, a large amount of muscle mass and muscle size, and a medium to high metabolism.

When you're an endomorph, you have a larger bone structure, a higher percentage of body fat, a smaller amount of muscle mass and muscle size, and a slow metabolism.

To reinforce this concept I suggest that you take a recent picture of yourself and one of your parents and grandparents when they were about your age. Compare the way all of you are built. A lot of what makes up your physique comes from their genes—you can't fight genetics! Big bones don't evolve into delicate bird bones. And if you're 5 feet 2 inches at age fifteen, you're never going to be 5 feet 11 inches. Long and lanky is not going to happen—but this doesn't make you an elf either. You're just petite. Some of you will grow up to have long legs and short waists, some of you will grow up to have short legs and long waists, and some of you will grow up to be equally proportioned.

While body type is something you're born with and can't necessarily change, you can change your eating habits and up your level of physical activity to decrease your body fat. Never forget that you can firm, tone, define, and enhance what you already have through fitness. Fitness is always a positive way of dealing with everything. It also provides a great release from the mental and emotional frustrations that come with being a teen.

avoid the enemy: your scale!

Scales are probably one of the worst inventions man ever designed. If the sight of yours makes you grimace, put it in your closet—or better yet, throw it away! Why? It's not an accurate gauge of your fitness level or your weight.

There is so much change in your growth between the ages of eleven and fifteen, including bones, muscles, internal organs—except for your lymphatic system (which actually decreases in size) and your brain, which reaches its maximum weight during your early teens. When, how, and how much these changes happen will vary with each of you and are determined by both your heredity and your environment. Around the age of eighteen, you could still grow another half inch. So of course you're going to get bigger during these years—it's expected!

One way to judge your size, without weighing yourself, is by how your clothes fit. If your height is not increasing, but your tops and bottoms are starting to feel snug, you need to consume less calories and expend more energy. Add your willpower and it's that simple. It will take 3,500 calories to gain a pound and a decrease of 3,500 calories to lose a pound.

There are several myths and misunderstandings about what fat is and isn't. As you increase your fitness level, consider the following:

1. Fat can be turned into muscle and muscle can be turned into fat. Not true! Muscle is a tissue and fat is a substance.

2. Muscle, which is lean body mass, weighs close to 75 percent more than fat. This means you can increase your weight, actually become leaner, and decrease your size.

3. You can tell if you're losing body fat, while you're working on toning and firming, by looking in the mirror with no clothes on. Be open-minded, and don't allow the mirror to intimidate you!

let's talk
about "healthy"

You know you can't change your body type, you've thrown away your scale, you're working on making the mirror your friend, and your main goal is fitness—right? So is there a way to judge if you are in a healthy range weight for your height? Yes, there is and it's one of my favorite tools, as it allows for your unique frame size and height. It's called the Body Mass Index, and it will clearly show you whether you're anorexic, underweight, healthy, overweight, or obese.

In order to find your Body Mass Index (BMI) you'll need to take everything off, know what your true weight and height are, and get out your calculator. This is also one time you will need a scale. I recommend that girls stop by their doctor's office and use that scale for accuracy. The doctor's scale also includes a height stick. Here's your formula (my example is a 5 feet 5 inches teen who weighs 130 pounds):

1. Divide your weight in pounds by 2.2 to get your weight in kilograms.

(Example: 130 lbs. / 2.2 = 59 kilograms)

2. Divide your height in inches by 39.4 to get your height in meters.

(Example: 5 feet 5 inches is 65 inches. So your computation is 65/ 39.4 = 1.65 meters.)

3. Square this number.

(Example: 1.65 x 1.65 = 2.72)

4. Now divide your weight number by your height number that's been squared. This gives you your BMI.

(Example: 59 kilograms / 2.72 = 21.7 BMI)

What are the ranges from anorexic to obese?

Anorexic = 16 or less

Underweight = 16–19

Healthy = 19–25

Overweight = 25–35

Obese = over 35

At 21.7, this BMI indicates the healthy range.

As you can see, this formula allows for a realistic latitude within each category. You'll also want to consider your own unique body and metabolism. Now, taking all of this into account, you should have a better idea of your fitness range.

seven tips to boost your self-esteem

Before we move on, I'd like to share with you seven tips that will boost your self-esteem. These are tips I offer my clients, who are really down on the way they look and feel, even before we start working on their fitness goals. Copy them and tape them to your mirror!

1. **What you see in the mirror is far less important when you look deep within yourself.** Peace of mind is the most important gift you can give yourself. Being happy from within gives you an external glow that can't be beat!

2. **See yourself as unique and fall in love with your looks.** This means accepting the fact that nobody, and I mean *nobody*, is perfect. Accentuate your best physical qualities and play up what makes you unique.

3. Wear your own skin—and wear it well! Forget about society's narrow-minded attitude of beauty. Be comfortable in your own skin. You don't have to measure up to anyone's standards.

4. Dressing for you is the best way to maintain your uniqueness. Who wants to be a second-rate imitation of anyone else? Individuality is always better than imitation. If you allow it, clothes can become just superficial garments that say nothing about who you really are.

5. No comparison shopping. This is another way of me telling you that you should never compare yourself to someone else. Thoughts of, "I don't measure up, my butt's not as small as hers, my boobs should be bigger, my waist should . . ." will make you project a negative self-image. You really do wear what you feel on the inside.

6. Focus on the ways that you can have an active, healthy routine and be grateful for the wonderful machine your body is! Fitness is not a penance. It's about being your personal best and having goals.

7. Your enthusiasm for life is the best drug there is for looking good and feeling good. It's 100 percent effective, totally natural, has no side effects, and is absolutely free. It's yours for the taking.

Eventually you will get older, and my wish for you is that you will think of your body as a road map of your life's special experiences. Not only can you learn to like your lines, but love them for what they mean to you—like the stretch marks that come in varying degrees from the miracle of giving birth. Each one of mine reminds me of my wonderful sons. The oldest are twins, so you can imagine what that did to me!

I know it's a personal choice, but I pray that you avoid the plastic surgeon's office because you loathe your boobs, your unique nose, you want to have the fat sucked out of your butt, or you want to erase time. Personally, I think a perfect body equates a shallow life. This doesn't include someone who has a great-looking body because of the gene pool—she just got the luck of the draw! For 95 percent of us it's going to mean working on our fitness levels. It can be lots of fun if you approach it with the right attitude.

I believe that if all you're concerned about is having a perfect body, then there's a lot of shallowness that exists within you. There are so many other aspects of life to nurture and cultivate. These are the things that you can enhance and that will only become more profound with age and experience, and therefore never leave you. Even the simplest things, like working on your smile and having an upbeat attitude, no matter how bad things get, count for a lot.

If the best body possible is what you're striving for, then at least do it the right way by challenging yourself and making gains in physical fitness. The end result may be that you get a look that you like, that *you find perfect*. I can respect those of you who do something concrete to get there.

The bottom line? Remember that a mirror is nothing more than a piece of glass that is easily shattered.

chapter three

Nutrition

Basics

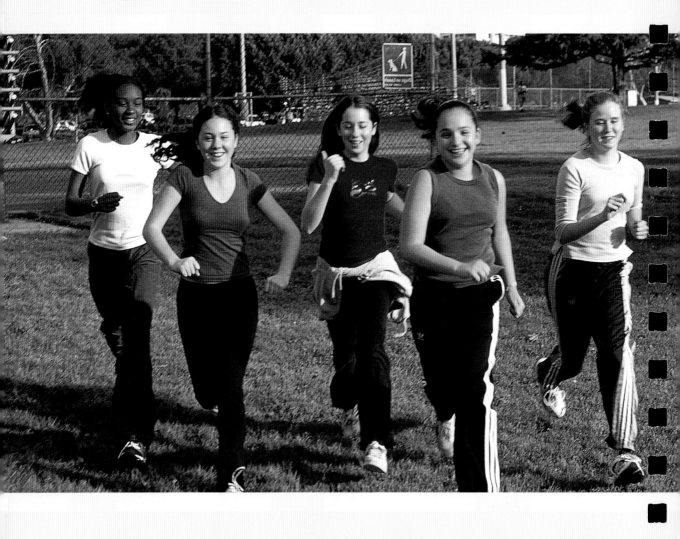

no permanent change happens overnight

Well, you know bingeing, purging, and starvation are all bad nutritional choices. In fact, you actually need to eat to lose. If you don't, you'll really mess up your metabolism—more about how and why later. So, how do you eat and reach a weight (really the BMI that I explained in the previous chapter) that's best for you? The best advice I can give you is to start slowly with all the nutritional information I'm about to share with you. You can't change your eating habits overnight. So, little by little, start incorporating some of the principles and tips in this chapter into your life. Stick with them, and I guarantee your eating habits will change. Start with one or two and add another every couple of days or every week until you're using all of them on a daily basis.

understanding the six necessary nutrition basics

All the foods we eat are made up of various combinations of the six basic food nutrients: carbohydrates, fats, proteins, vitamins, minerals, and water. Carbohydrates, fats, and proteins seem to be the most controversial these days, so let's examine why they're essential in our diet:

Carbohydrates are a primary source of energy for the cells in our bodies—brain cells and muscle cells. The carb family includes complex carbohydrates such as potatoes, oatmeal, white and brown rice, yams, and all varieties of bread. The carb family also includes fruit, as well as simple sugars, including soda pop, table sugar, baked goods, and candy. The body converts all the carbs we eat into glucose, which the cells then convert into energy. Today, most experts recommend that we get 60 to 65 percent of our daily calories from complex carbohydrates.

Fats, like carbs, come in two major groups: saturated and unsaturated. The main purpose of fat is energy production. We don't need to eat very much fat of any kind. About 20 to 25 percent of our daily calories is the normal recommendation. *Fat is not bad*. And yes, our bodies need some—but not too much.

Proteins are used mainly for providing the structure for the many cells and tissues in our bodies. They are also used in the immune system and to make up many of our hormones. Like insulin, protein is a vital part of our body, but we don't need a lot of it. Ten to 15 percent of our daily calories is the general recommendation.

Along with following the appropriate exercise program, my clients have great success losing weight when they eat a balanced diet (all of the above) in moderation. We never call it *dieting*.

basic meal planning

Breakfast, lunch, a snack or two, and dinner is your ideal daily meal plan. When you eat like this, your body is fueled throughout your busy day. Unfortunately, during the week a traditional breakfast is rarely feasible. Many of you have parents (and some both!) who are out the door, rushing off to work, while you're still getting dressed.

This is tough when you're going to school, because you have to take responsibility for your breakfast (it really is the best way to start the day)—but who wants to think about eating so early in the morning, especially if you hate breakfast?!

if you hate breakfast . . .

These are easy ways to get fruit in your diet, as well as something nutritious to fill you up before you leave for school:

Chilean Glacier Whirl

(In case you're wondering, "Chilean" means fruit from Chile. In fact, except for citrus fruits, all of our fruits and vegetables come from Chile during the winter because Chile is in its summer season when we're in our winter season.) In a blender put the following ingredients and blend on high for 15 seconds. Delicious!

1 Chilean nectarine or peach, cut into chunks
½ cup milk
½ cup orange juice
1 tbsp. honey
¼ tsp. almond extract
2 ice cubes

Kathy's Favorite Shake

Blend this up—yum! This is what I like to have before leaving in the morning.

1 handful frozen fresh strawberries (When I get strawberries at the store I just wash them, take the stems off, and put them in a zipped freezer bag.)
1 cup vanilla-flavored soy milk
Splash of orange juice
½ banana (the other half I eat later)

If you don't have time to sit down to a bowl of granola, or other high-fiber cereal you like, a bran muffin, a bagel, or a piece of whole wheat toast (topped with a little cream cheese or a splash of jelly), and a piece of fresh fruit are also tasty breakfast alternatives. Hard-boiled eggs are good too. You can take any of these "to go." Try to avoid sweets. The sugar high that comes with sweet rolls or dough-nuts is not the way to begin your day. Within two hours you'll start feeling sluggish.

Given the quality of most cafeteria food, many teens have told me that lunch can be a real nightmare. Often by the time they actually get to the food, the lunch period is over. I suggest that you pack your lunch—if not in the morning, then the night before—and refrigerate it.

A sandwich, veggies, and a piece of fruit should get you through the rest of your school day. Make up tuna or egg salad and refrigerate it in a small container. You can avoid a soggy sandwich by wrapping the whole-grain bread separately. All of it, with a small bottle of water, can go in a nifty little thermal lunch bag. You can buy one in almost any discount store that sells lunch boxes, thermoses, backpacks, camping supplies, and the like.

An all-time after-school snack favorite is salted, air-popped pop-corn. There's no fat involved (unless you add melted butter), it has lots of fiber, and may be the next best thing to chips. Sorbet and low-fat ice cream are good too—just don't polish off an entire carton.

It's so easy for your exhausted parents to pick up fast food for din-ner. Urge them not to. Now may be a good time in your life to begin experimenting with cooking. Get the cookbooks out and be creative! If there are none in the house, check out the bookstores; there is such a variety to choose from that offer all kinds of well-balanced, tasty recipes. You'll learn a lot about food, and even more about the different food groups that are coming up.

what about specific diets?

I'm sure that you have heard about a "zillion" different diets since you've become body conscious, which usually starts when puberty begins. You've seen them advertised on TV and in magazines, and numerous books have been written about them—books that have actually made the *New York Times* best-seller list. I could scream! Fad diets never work in the long haul, and they have the potential to damage your body.

A long time ago, I watched Richard Simmons on television, cheering everyone on about losing weight and sweating, as he started to talk about diets. He told the host to look at the first three letters in that word—*D I E*—and then he asked, "Who wants to die?"

What he said has stuck with me for a long time. You do suffer on any kind of diet. You already have enough pressure to deal with just by being a teenager. Now you're putting restrictions on yourself, which creates additional pressure and makes you feel bad, because no one feels good about themselves when they're on a diet.

I know people who have tried every diet they've heard about. The end result? They're fatter than they were before.

Traditionally, diets demand that you reduce your caloric intake. The message your body gets is that it's not going to be getting enough fuel. Automatically, your body metabolism slows itself down to save all the energy it can. Since it doesn't know when it's going to be fed again, saving fat is the only thing your body knows to do. You continue to diet, you will lose lean muscle mass, but you will increase the amount of body fat you have. When you've had enough of the deprivation, most likely you will resume your old eating habits, and boom—you gain weight again!

Some people call it yo-yo dieting. I call it a vicious cycle. You gain and lose and gain and lose, all the while increasing the amount of body fat you have.

Many of the diet best-sellers not only do what I just explained, but also have significant health risks. Some recommend that if you cut out entire food groups, carbohydrates for example, you will lose a lot of weight within weeks. What you're not told is that challenging the balance of your nutrients can have damaging effects on your body. You can become constipated, dehydrated, and sluggish. Your kidneys may go into overdrive from too much protein, which could cause harm.

Eventually, you will tire of all the protein, stop the diet, and gain back the weight you've lost, which is probably mostly water anyway. You think it's worth jeopardizing your health for this? I don't think so. In all the years that I've been a fitness trainer, I don't think I've observed anyone doing well when they're being restricted—it only creates cravings and obsessions.

So what's the answer? Moderation in food balanced with exercise. For instance, if you're having a submarine sandwich, eat just half of it instead of the whole thing. Don't buy "fat free" cookies, which will tempt you to eat half of the box. Instead, stop by the bakery and buy one fresh-baked cookie. Enjoy every morsel—but one is all!

Remember, if you need to lose (whether you're a teen or an adult), for every pound you want to drop, you're going to have to use up 3,500 calories. This means cutting back on high-calorie foods and exercising more. Notice I didn't mention deprivation or diet—you just have to change your eating and exercise habits. The same is true if you need to gain, only in reverse—but don't stop exercising. (No one should ever stop exercising unless they are sick or have an injury that needs to heal.) Just start slowly increasing your caloric levels.

calories and you

Should you be "counting calories"? I don't think so, but it doesn't hurt to be aware that certain foods are very high in fat and calories, while others are very low. For instance, a handful of cashews contains a lot more calories than a handful of grapes.

During this time in your life, your body is growing in so many different ways—and its growth comes in spurts. You may find yourself ravenous during these spurts, so you need the extra fuel. At other times, maintain the healthy moderation I've been talking about.

nineteen terrific eating tips to get you through your day

1. Don't skip breakfast. Make yourself sit down, then try a bowl of cereal with low-fat milk, a glass of juice, a piece of whole wheat toast with a fruit spread. Don't be surprised when your grades improve and you feel more energized throughout the day! If you're not hungry in the morning, you will be if you stop eating three hours before you go to bed. Sometimes you are not hungry in the morning because you've made it a habit not to eat.

2. Eat a serving of something that is red and orange. Eating "colors" means you're getting lots of different kinds of minerals and vitamins (a handful of red grapes, strawberries, raspberries, an orange, a sweet potato, a cup of cantaloupe, red bell peppers, sliced tomatoes).

3. When you are about to snack on something, ask yourself if you are really hungry.

4. Get three servings of calcium a day. This is a must, and I'll tell you why later in this chapter. (Here are some choices: skimmed or low-fat milk, yogurt, cottage cheese, or orange juice fortified with calcium.)

5. Drink lots of water throughout the day. Pour yourself 8 to 10 glasses a day. Place water bottles around the house wherever you're going to be. Most schools, especially in hot climates like California, allow plastic water bottles. If your school doesn't, try to get at least 2 glasses in at lunchtime.

6. With two of your meals add something that is green. Green provides you with different vitamins than purple, red, and orange. (Some examples: broccoli, green beans, asparagus, green peppers, or spinach.)

7. When you snack, go for lower-fat choices like pretzels, air-popped popcorn, sorbet, frozen fruit bars, pita chips with salsa, English muffin with a fruit spread, raisins, or fruit.

8. If you drink diet soda, make a deal with yourself: before you have a can, you must drink 2 of your 8 to 10 glasses of water.

9. If you are a fast-food junkie—tacos, fries, chili dogs, dough-nuts—and eat these at least once a day, start cutting back one day a week and find a healthier choice. After a week, cut back two days and eat at a healthier place. Continue until you're down to one day of junk food a week—better yet, one day a month.

10. Walk around the block before you eat a snack. By the time you've finished your walk, you may no longer want the snack.

11. If you're at a restaurant, order what you want, but ask that it be

broiled or grilled. If it's something very high in fat and calories, ask for an appetizer size.

12. Try eating a well-balanced breakfast, make lunch your main meal of the day, and have a small dinner. If the lunch choice offered at school doesn't balance out your nutritional needs, pack your own lunch.

13. Eat until you're no longer hungry, not until you're full.

14. Ask Mom to keep a bowl of cut-up vegetables and fruit in the refrigerator for snacks. This way you're sure to get several servings of fruits and vegetables a day. If she's too busy, there's no reason you can't fix these for yourself.

15. Double up on fruit. Most of us only get half of what we need. As a teen you need at least two servings a day. I recommend four servings. One serving is usually ½ cup. Examples: a handful of grapes, 1 apple, ½ sliced melon.

    You may have heard that fruit is high in sugar. However, this is a natural sugar called *fructose* and is the best form of a simple carbohydrate because it contains vitamins, minerals, and fiber. Conversely, baked goods, sweets, and candy are full of a refined sugar called *sucrose* and don't provide any nutritional value.

16. Ask Mom and Dad to keep chips and treats out of the house.

17. It only takes 75 to 100 calories to satisfy your sweet tooth. So take your favorite candy bar, cut it up into thirds, freeze two pieces of them, and eat just one. This way you have two left for your next two sweet attacks.

18. Don't fall for the fat-free sweet frenzy. Just because something is fat free doesn't mean it's not loaded with sugar calories.

19. I recommend that you take a multivitamin daily. It's not a substitute for good food, but it may help give you extra protection during the cold and flu season.

water, water, water

Water is the best thing that you can drink. In fact, you can never get enough of it, and there are no limitations on how much you should drink as long as you are healthy.

Water, which makes up about 60 percent of the average person's body composition, is vital in sustaining normal body functions and overall health. It aids in digestion, blood production, and breathing. It also helps solid waste move through your intestines. Without water in your body, you would poison yourself. It lubricates your joints, keeping you limber. And water helps regulate your body temperature. When you work out or are really hot, you naturally start sweating to cool down. That sweat comes from the water in your body.

The jury is still out on the best water to drink, because there are so many kinds available. Many health experts recommend that you drink bottled water from the purest sources, high mountain ranges far from urban areas, glacial waters, and the deep artesian wells of Fiji. As far as I'm concerned, just drink any kind of water and as much as possible—regardless of the brand! When it comes to tap water, I recommend that you boil it first (because of the chemicals in it), let it cool, and then put it in plastic bottles. If you're concerned about the potential toxicity of your tap water, you can contact the Environmental Protection Agency Safe Drinking Water Hotline at (800) 426-4791 for the scoop on what's coming out of your faucet.

So how much water do you need to drink? Well, I know you've heard at least eight 8-ounce glasses a day—but do you really get that? Try not to include any other kind of liquid. Juices, coffees, teas, sodas, and beer do not count. These drinks may contain sugar, chemicals, caffeine, and alcohol, and some of them dehydrate you. Did you know that a good portion of the population is living in a state of partial dehydration?

If you are used to drinking everything but water, start carrying a bottle with you. It's not only a trendy thing to do—it's a necessary thing to do! Leave big bottles in the car, keep a bottle next to your bed. Get in the habit of drinking water with your meal. A glass of water before you eat can make you feel a little full and help you cut down on overeating.

Drinking water cleanses the inside of your body. And wait until you see what it does for your skin! Don't be surprised when you start having fewer breakouts.

When you exercise, you must pay attention to your water needs. A workout in warm weather could drain as much as 7 quarts of water from your body. This is why you should drink water before, during, and after exercise.

You can be creative with your water. Freeze some lemon juice in an ice cube tray and drop one cube into a big glass of water. It gives you just a bit of flavor and a bit of fun. Buy yourself a really beautiful or silly glass. If it's unique and you know it's special, it may get you to drink a few extra glasses. I know this works for me.

Drink sodas in moderation because they're filled either with sugar or chemicals. If I have not had enough water during the day, I don't feel that I've earned a soda.

Juice is a good choice, because it gives you additional vitamins and minerals. But it also gives you a lot of extra calories, which is why I only drink it sparingly. One day my twin boys taught me a neat trick at the kitchen table: they were playing with cups of water and diluting it with their juice. Of course I had to taste-test it before they'd let me out the door—and it was great. You still get the taste of juice, but with half the calories!

Another trick is that I'm never without a case of water in my car. Since I'm on the road a lot going to train clients, I play a game with myself. I have to drink one whole bottle before I reach my destination.

To start upping your water intake, begin your day with a glass of water. Have another glass before breakfast and, whenever possible, drink it at school. Have a glass before your snack after school, another glass before dinner, a glass during dinner, and a glass while you're watching television. That's at least 7 glasses right there. And of course, as I already said, you'll be drinking water before, during, and after you exercise.

Remember, think to drink. And if you can't remember, do what my one friend's fifteen-year-old daughter does: she writes WATER on the palm of each hand.

dairy in your diet means calcium for life

The calcium you get from the foods you eat and the milk you drink as a child and as a teenager profoundly affects your bone strength and bone density now and for the rest of your life. Calcium is so important in your diet that you could almost consider it a separate food group.

You build the majority of your bone density during adolescence. This is when your body works most efficiently to deposit bone-building calcium in your bones. When you don't get enough calcium during this crucial time, and really up to the age of thirty, you risk ending up with bones that become extremely porous as you get older. You could develop osteoporosis, a brittle bone disease that leads to easy-to-fracture bones and possibly a permanent, stooped-over posture.

Sound scary? It is, and many younger women are now at risk because they've purposely avoided dairy products due to the misconception that they're fattening. Consequently, 88 percent of all teenage girls do not meet current calcium recommendations.

Ironically, recent studies show that a diet that contains low-fat dairy products may actually help you lose weight as it burns body fat. Apparently, dairy's antiobesity effects are largely due to its high calcium content as well as something else that hasn't been identified yet. I know this sounds strange, but as I write this scientists still don't have a reason for why it happens.

Osteoporosis is responsible for 1.5 million fractures annually, including 500,000 vertebral fractures and more than 300,000 hip fractures. In fact, a woman's lifetime risk of dying from complications after a hip fracture is about the same as her lifetime risk of dying from breast cancer—about one in eight.

The good news is that it is preventable! Throughout your life, a diet rich in calcium, vitamin D, which helps your body absorb calcium from food and deposit the mineral into your bones, and regular weight-bearing exercise will do the trick. Why weight-bearing exercise? This kind of activity, including brisk walking, jogging, racquet sports, and aerobic dancing, stimulates bone formation.

Between the ages of nine and eighteen you need to consume the greatest amount of calcium a day—at least 1,300 milligrams. Regardless of the type of milk you choose—whole, low-fat, or fat-free—it is one of the best sources of calcium. Eight ounces will meet 300 milligrams of your daily requirement of calcium.

8 OUNCES	CALORIES	FAT	CALCIUM
whole milk	150	8 gm.	291 mg.
2% reduced-fat milk	120	5 gm.	297 mg.
1% low-fat milk	102	3 gm.	300 mg.
fat-free milk	86	0 gm.	302 mg.

If you don't like milk, try mixing it with bananas or berries and ice in a blender for a homemade smoothie. Also, you can exchange your 8-ounce glass of milk for:

- 8 ounces of yogurt
- 8 ounces of buttermilk
- 1½ ounces of natural cheese
- 1 cup of pudding
- 1½ cups of frozen yogurt
- 2 cups of cottage cheese
- 1½ cups of ice cream
- 1 cup of macaroni and cheese
- 4½ ounces of canned salmon
- 1½ cups of okra
- 1 cup of collard greens
- 8 ounces of tofu (made with calcium)
- 3 cups of broccoli
- 6 oranges
- 6 corn tortillas

reading labels

Whether you're a teen or an adult, how to read labels on packaged food products is one of the most valuable things you can learn. Knowing what's in anything packaged that you eat, including the basics—protein grams, carb grams, and fat percentage—will help you become and remain nutritionally fit. Manufacturers are now required to put a nutritional label on almost all food products.

When you learn the percentage of fat calories in a particular item, it will help you plan your snacks and meals for the rest of the day, because each fat gram has more calories than protein or carbohydrates.

But be aware of the "marketing myth" that because a food is low in fat, fat-free, or sugar-free, you can consume unlimited quantities. This is not true! Any food eaten in excess of the calories you've burned in a day will be stored as body fat. When you read the label, look for the caloric content as well as the fat calories per serving. Also, pay attention to the number of servings offered. Two servings at 90 calories each is equal to 180 calories if you consume the entire product.

I have one client who was thrilled when she realized that while potato chips had about 50 percent fat calories, yogurt had none. Immediately, she assumed that she could eat as much yogurt as she wanted because there was no fat in it. Not only was she perplexed when she didn't lose weight—but totally confused when she actually gained two pounds. I had to burst her bubble and remind her that yogurt still had 100 calories per serving. Bottom line was that the energy balance relationship still remains the same, regardless of where the calories come from.

THE NUTRITION FACTS FOOD LABEL

NUTRITION FACTS

Serving Size 1 cup (228 g)
Servings Per Container 2

AMOUNT PER SERVING

Calories 260   Calories from Fat 120

	% daily values
Total Fat 13g	20%
Saturated Fat 5g	25%
Cholesterol 30mg	10%
Sodium 660 mg	28%
Total Carbohydrate 31g	10%
Dietary Fiber 0g	0%
Sugars 5g	
Protein 5g	

· Vitamin A 4%   · Vitamin C 2%
· Calcium 15%   · Iron 4%

Percent Daily Values are based on a 2000 calorie diet.
Your daily values may be higher or lower depending on
your calorie needs:

	Calories:	2000	2500
Total Fat	Less than	65g	80g
Saturated Fat	Less than	20g	25g
Cholesterol	Less than	300mg	300mg
Sodium	Less than	2,400mg	2,400mg
Total Carbohydrate		300g	375g
Dietary Fiber		25g	30g

Calories per gram:
Fat 9 · Carbohydrate 4 · Protein 4

SERVING SIZE
The serving size for this food is one cup. All the nutrition numbers listed are based on this amount. Compare the serving size to the amount you eat and adjust the numbers as needed. For example if you ate two cups of this food, you'd double the numbers shown (e.g., 520 calories).

SERVINGS PER CONTAINER
Note carefully! Even small packages sometimes contain more than one serving. This package contains two servings.

NUTRITION NUMBERS
The label lists the number of calories and the number of Calories from Fat in one serving. Also listed are the grams of Total Fat, Saturated Fat, Total Carbohydrate, Dietary Fiber, Sugars, Protein and miligrams of Cholesteral and Sodium.

PERCENT DAILY VALUES
These percents show how much of each nutrient one serving provides in a 2,000-calorie diet. For the label shown here, one serving of food provides 20% of the Total Fat and 15% of the Calcium recommended for the day.

HIT YOUR TARGETS
For nutrients we sometimes get too much of (Fat, Saturated Fat, Cholesterol, and Sodium), your daily goal is to total 100% or less of the Daily Value. For Nutrients such as Calcium, Iron, Vitamin A, and Vitamin C, your daily goal is to reach 100% of the Daily Value. Reading the label helps you balance out your food choices. For example, you can balance out higher fat foods with lower fat foods so you don't exceed your daily target.

To figure out the number of calories per serving:

Protein: the amount of the product that is protein is usually stated in grams. Multiply the number of grams listed (per serving) by 4. This gives you the number of calories per serving.

Carbohydrate: the amount of the product that is carbohydrate is also stated in grams. Multiply the number of grams listed (per serving) by 4. This gives you the number of calories per serving.

Fat: the amount of the product that is fat is usually stated in grams. However, each fat gram gives you a higher number of calories. Instead of multiplying the number by 4, as you do for protein and carbs, multiply the number of grams listed (per serving) by 9. This gives you the number of calories per serving.

The more label reading you do, the more useful it will become. It will help you maximize calcium intake and minimize fat intake. You will learn how you can get more food per day, while losing weight or just maintaining where you are. You will also learn more about the other vitamins and minerals that you are going to need, like vitamin C and iron.

don't let pms get the better of you

As if the bloating, irritability, fatigue, and depression weren't enough, with PMS usually comes an intense craving for junk food that is sweet and salty. I know girls who would live on fries, potato chips, candy, and chocolate ice cream for that week before their period begins. Besides the fact that these foods have little nutritional value, they only make your PMS worse.

Salty foods can make you more bloated than you already are, and sugar can make you more tired and depressed once the high has worn off. Both of these contribute to your tiny blemishes blowing up into puffy pimples.

Instead of going for the junk, reach for fresh fruits, veggies, whole-grain products, and low-salt/low-sugar food. Once your period has passed, you'll thank yourself for not giving in to temptation. Here are some PMS concoctions that should subdue your irrational cravings:

- scooped-out bagel filled with low-fat cottage cheese or low-fat cream cheese
- fruit smoothies
- baked fries
- toast with peanut butter
- papaya wedges with lime
- baked apple
- baked sweet potato wedges
- low-salt pretzels

Also, don't forget to drink lots of water!!! It will clean the excess salt out of your system that is apt to collect at this time.

eating during parties, movies, and dates

According to nutritionist Elizabeth Ward, you should never go to a movie, party, or out on a date starving. Before you leave the house, have a big glass of low-fat milk, a hard-boiled egg, or even another fruit shake.

At the movies, it's easy to polish off a bucket of popcorn that's been popped in oil. Instead, go for the smallest size and a diet soda.

If you're craving candy, bring a small box of your own: Junior Mints, licorice, jelly beans, or gumdrops. They're sweet and provide little or no fat. (They have lots of calories, though.)

At parties, avoid the chips and dips if possible. Look for celery, carrots, and cheese cubes. Go for a half slice of pizza instead of a whole one. If your boyfriend or date is still hungry after the party and wants junk food, suggest healthy junk. Let him order the burger and fries while you head for the salad bar.

I'm the first to admit that it's easy to indulge when you're surrounded by food. Again, it's all about moderation, and remembering your fitness goals. But I don't want you beating yourself up if you fall off the wagon. This is how eating disorders begin. Remember, you can always resume the good habits that you've been developing, tomorrow.

chapter four

Eating Properly and Breaking Bad Habits

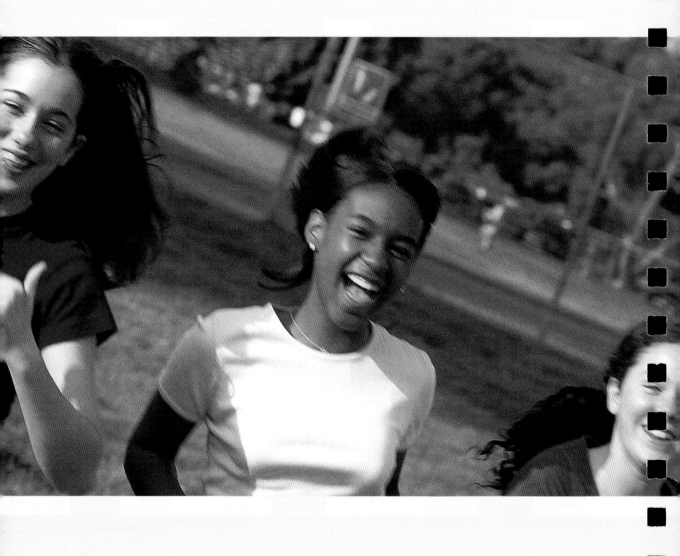

Over the years I've learned a lot about breaking bad habits, which can prevent any of us from eating properly, from my own mistakes. Obviously, nutritional needs will vary depending upon your health and fitness goals.

Don't be surprised if even minor changes in your eating habits lead to a much healthier diet. Much of the following advice I've learned from the best in the fitness and nutrition field. Setting good habits now, in your teens, means that you are on a path to fitness and ideally no unmanageable weight problems for the rest of your life.

the side effects of not eating properly

If you experience any of the following symptoms, your body may be warning you that you're losing too much weight or missing certain necessary nutrients:

Constant Fatigue. What's missing: complex carbohydrates (pasta, rice, beans, potatoes). Also, skipping meals lowers blood sugar and drains energy.

Dry, Dull Skin; Brittle Nails. What's missing: protein, iron, and vitamins B_6 and B_{12} (all found in lean meats)—and folic acid (found in leafy greens and orange juice). These nutrients are needed for the blood's oxygen transport.

Changes in Taste or Smell. What's missing: you need zinc, which is bountiful in meat and seafood.

Bad Breath. You're missing liquids, especially water, which rinse your mouth of odor-producing bacteria.

Cuts and Bruises That Don't Heal. What's missing: antioxidants (beta-carotene and vitamins E and C), which are plentiful in fruits and vegetables.

Feeling Cold All the Time; Lack of Menstruation; Stress Fractures. Believe it or not, you need fat and calories! This can indicate an eating disorder, or one that's beginning to develop.

flipping the
food pyramid

Most food pyramids have the tip at the top, or what you should eat in the smallest quantities. I have always inverted the pyramid, focusing on the positive, reinforcing what you can eat in abundance. As for the tip, which is now on the bottom and contains the sweets, fats, and junk food, I say, "Indulge sparingly—but enjoy every bite!"

Bread, Cereal, Rice
and Pasta Group
(6–11 servings)

Vegetable Group
(3–5 servings)

Fruit Group
(2–4 servings)

Milk, Yogurt, and
Cheese Group
(2–3 servings)

Meat, Poultry,
Fish, Dry Beans,
Eggs, and
Nuts Group
(2–3 servings)

Fats and Sweets
(use sparingly)

the 90-10 principle

The 90-10 principle is something I learned when I was working in Colorado at a health club. I was working in the wellness center with my friend Dr. Daniel Kosich. He had developed a program called Fatburners. An important part of his program was the 90-10 principle. It works so well that I have since used this as a way of life, and I share it with all of my clients. Basically, it's a way of thinking.

> Slow down. Eat slowly enough that your body knows that you are eating. Count to 10 with each bite. I have made my husband do this with me. It has helped him feel fuller and less hungry later on in the evening.

While losing weight, many people tell themselves they can never eat certain foods again. I'm the perfect example. I love chocolate. Now, if I were to tell myself that I couldn't have it, this would make me crazy. So crazy, in fact, that I would obsess over it, and the next time I saw chocolate, I would buy two bars instead of one and eat it all. After that last, delicious bite, I would feel as if I had no self-control. My self-esteem would take a nosedive because I'd eaten this "bad" food.

You should never label your food as "good" or "bad." In fact, I would try to stay away from positive or negative labels altogether. These labels make you feel worse about yourself and deprived. Eventually, you are going to start feeling bad about yourself and eat even more of your "bad" food.

The best way to counteract this problem is to think positively about all food. Food is a wonderful thing. We live in a country where we are blessed with an abundance of quality food. It is how we eat this food that counts.

Now this is where the 90-10 principle comes in. Ninety percent of the time I eat well. This means lots of fruits, vegetables, and whole grains. I buy lean meat and watch the fat. I consume less simple sugar carbohydrates and more high complex carbohydrates. And, I always drink plenty of water.

The 10 percent takes place when I want something that may not fit into these categories, because it has a lot of sugar, is full of fat, or contains a lot of calories, or just tastes awesome. Ideally, I save my 10 percent for special occasions, such as weddings, family gatherings, parties, or a vacation.

If I'm really having a craving, sometimes the 10 percent is eaten on a weekly basis, a daily basis—or even on a meal basis. But I toe the line when it comes to not going over the 10 percent mark.

I like pizza, chocolate, and high-fat cheese. They definitely all fall into the 10 percent category. When I do have any of these, I

> Eat more foods that are high in complex carbohydrates. These include rice, cereal, whole-grain bread, pastas, beans, fruits, and vegetables. They have more fiber, which fills you up, and they contain less calories too—although you should still be aware of the size of your portions and the amount, if any, of the sauces, dressings, and butter that you add.

> You can curb your appetite by drinking a big glass of water before any meal. This will help you feel full.

just make sure during the same day that I have fruits, vegetables, protein, and good carbohydrates. A lot depends on what is happening in my life. And that is something none of us has any control over.

Life. A lot of things come up that are unexpected. If you have complicated and restrictive dietary habits, you are going to have a tough time. That's why I think the 90-10 eating principle is a reasonable way to deal with any lifestyle. I might pig out for one night, but I know tomorrow I can resume my 90-10 eating way of life. It works, allows you to maintain your Body Mass Index, and it's something you can live with for the rest of your life.

what kind of eater are you?

Everyone has an eating style. Here are some tips that will help you maximize your nutrition and utilize the 90-10 principle, regardless of your style.

Here a Meal, There a Meal. You have so much going on that you often forget to eat until your stomach growls so loud that everyone around you can hear. While your friends may think you're lucky not to be obsessed about food, going too long without food can lead to energy depletion. You also may be missing vitamins, minerals, and other nutrients your body needs. So make it a point to fuel your body regularly by trying the following:

- Don't leave your house without having breakfast. Have a banana (or another favorite fruit) and a bagel or some yogurt. Or a warm bowl of oatmeal made with milk and topped with fruit is a great way to start your day.
- Pack some healthy snacks the night before so that you can refuel every three hours while you're on the go: an apple, an orange, string cheese, trail mix, and whole wheat crackers. Don't forget your water!
- Make time for a sit-down dinner with your family as often as you can. It's fun to play catch-up and a great way to relieve a stressful day. If after-school sports or activities cause you to miss dinner, make sure you still sit down to a satisfying and nutritious meal.

Snack Attacker. You just can't understand the concept of three square meals a day. Reaching for whatever is handy, you'd rather snack at all hours. While your energy may stay sky-

Eat what you like. There is nothing worse than being told what to eat when it's something that you hate. Just remember that moderation is the key. This may take some willpower, but applying the 90-10 principle will help.

high, the same may be true for your calorie count if you choose chips, cookies, fries, and soda. Instead, reach for:

- Low-fat cheese and crackers, hummus and pita bread, raisin toast with a thin layer of peanut butter, or homemade soup. All of these contain carbs, protein, and fat, which satisfies your hunger longer. These should help you avoid reaching for that quick fix.
- Try getting into the meal mood. At least one balanced meal a day will help you get enough fruits and veggies.
- If you're a soda fiend, try replacing it with water, fat-free milk, or calcium-fortified O.J.

Eager Eater. You love food, and there's nothing wrong with that, so you're getting the nutrition you need. Your problem is that you may find your waistline expanding. Basically, you need to plan your attack on food! Think carefully before you make your first move:

- Think in terms of trade-offs. If you're going to dinner after the movies, avoid theater munchies. If you eat a big breakfast, try skipping your snack and have a light lunch—think salad!
- Be aware. Before you eat, ask yourself if you're eating because you're hungry or just because the food is there. Also, don't mistake hunger for thirst—drink a glass of water and wait ten minutes before you snack.
- Choose snacks wisely. It's easy to dig your hand into a box of cookies and start munching away. Before you realize it, you've eaten at least half a box or more.

fiber
fitness

Eating properly means including lots of fiber in your diet. Natural fiber sources are nutritious, good for your heart, and can help you lose weight in at least three ways:

1. Fiber expands in your belly, making you feel fuller on fewer calories.

2. High-fiber foods take a lot longer to chew than low-fiber ones, encouraging you to eat less. A good example is a hearty mixed-grain bread versus white bread. Or try eating a piece of celery quickly—impossible!

3. Fiber traps some of the fat you ingest from your food, moving it through your system before your body has the chance to absorb it all. Food high in fiber can also help

> Reward your fitness efforts with a shopping spree, a facial, or a free makeover at your local department store. It's important to pat yourself on the back as you make these healthy changes.
>
> When an eating plan tells you that you can lose more than two pounds per week, steer clear!

> Never eat directly from a carton, container, or package. You'll have no idea of the exact amount you're consuming. Make sure always to eat from bowls or plates unless you're having a premeasured, prepackaged snack.

prevent the bloating that can come with constipation, *but you must drink at least 8 glasses of water a day* to feel and see the benefit. If you don't drink enough water, the fiber could constipate you, because the excess bulk of the fiber can't pass through your digestive system.

The following foods are not only high in fiber, but are tasty too: almonds (and other nuts), apples with their peel, apricots, baked potatoes with their skin, bran, broccoli, Brussels sprouts, corn, kiwi fruit, oats, popcorn, raspberries, strawberries, and all whole-grain products.

> Eat colors. Focusing on colorful, nutritious food, try to eat as many colors as you can in one day, every day. Look for green, red, orange, purple, and yellow fruits and veggies.

skinny pizza

Who doesn't like pizza? A new survey reports that it's the number one choice for dinner, and that it can be a good choice too.

While restaurants serving pizza do differ in preparation, in general a mere two slices of the deluxe style with "the works" is about 750 calories and has 36 grams of fat. Fortunately, there are a lot of alternatives. To begin with, try eating just one slice instead of two, and have it with a big salad that includes chick peas and kidney beans. This fits in nicely with the 90-10 principle. Also, try out some of the slimming alternatives. Here are some options:

ONE SLICE OF	EQUALS
No-cheese veggie pizza	170 cal. and 7 gm. fat
Cheese pizza, extra-thin crust	205 cal. and 8 gm. fat
Mushroom pizza	210 cal. and 8 gm. fat
Pepperoni pizza	215 cal. and 10 gm. fat
Bacon pizza	220 cal. and 12 gm. fat
Extra-cheese pizza	225 cal. and 9 gm. fat
Regular cheese pizza	235 cal. and 9 gm. fat
Sausage pizza	235 cal. and 12 gm. fat
Cheese pizza, extra-thick crust	260 cal. and 11 gm. fat
Meat-topped pizza (with ham, sausage, bacon, etc.)	315 cal. and 11 gm. fat
Supreme pizza (stuffed crust, extra everything!)	375 cal and 18 gm. fat

the
pill-popping trap

How many advertisements have you seen or read where they're trying to get you to buy a pill to improve some aspect of your body, including your hair, nails, skin, teeth, and bones? Then there are pills to keep you from getting sick, pills to give you energy, pills to make you go to the bathroom—the list goes on and on. Companies that make these pills are generating billions of dollars a year off consumers.

Well, I'm not one of them.

Except when I was taking over-the-counter diet pills, I have never fallen into the pill-popping trap (only my daily multivitamin and a prenatal vitamin when I was pregnant). It's not a question whether or not they work. Rather, taking a pill to remedy a health issue does not teach you the valuable lessons of how to take care of yourself naturally. Of course if you're ill or in pain, you should follow your physician's advice.

In general, forget the pills and focus on improving the quality of your diet, and therefore your health, with variety. I think you know by now that I'm going to stress lots of

> Don't give up—even if you have a bad day or you experienced an event that got you off your health wagon. Get right back on. Your body doesn't respond that quickly for you to throw in the towel. Just recognize what's starting to happen and get back on track the next day.

fruits and vegetables in a variety of colors, whole grains, calcium-rich dairy products, and lean meats, chicken, and fish.

Your body responds better when it gets vitamins from natural sources—not a bottle. What could be better than getting your vitamin C directly from a big juicy orange?

Don't go vitamin crazy! I know people who take so many different ones in the morning that they have special containers to keep them in. Having had their vitamins, they eat horrible junk stuff all day long, but don't feel guilty because they've taken their vitamins. This just doesn't make sense to me—not to mention the monthly cost of all those pills!

stay off the coffee bandwagon

So what's wrong with drinking Java? For starters, it leaches that precious calcium you've been working so hard to store in your bones right out of those bones.

Today there are more coffeehouses than ever. These chic hot spots are popping up on every corner, and they have turned a cup of coffee into a gourmet drink brimming with excess calories. Add the cream, the mocha, the cremes, the different flavors—and you're drinking a meal. Not to mention never passing by the glass cases without getting something sweet to nibble on! If any of you visit these places habitually, you are probably not including these calories in your day and you wonder why you're putting on a little weight.

All of the above holds true for the new juice bars too. A juice smoothie may have as many calories as your breakfast and lunch combined.

I think the best way to go is with a bottle of your favorite water or a glass of nonfat milk. Both will quench your thirst, and one glass of nonfat milk will provide you with 300 milligrams of your daily calcium requirement—not to mention saving a few bucks!

you are what you eat

Have you ever looked at people you don't even know but can tell they aren't healthy? Their skin tone may be strange, their complexions poor, their hair dull, and they probably radiate very little energy. They don't look real. If you were to follow them through their daily routine, chances are good that every meal they ate would be fast food or processed junk food—they're eating "fake." And I don't think you'd see them drinking much water—probably a soda instead, like I used to, and diet soda at that!

Sometimes I'd have three sodas a day. This was when my eating disorder was really kicking in. I know now that the caffeine and the aspartame (artificial sweetener) I was consuming may have contributed to my seizure disorder as well as my downward nutritional spiral.

Limit your use of "diet" anything. Aspartame, also known as Equal and NutraSweet, is an extremely controversial additive in diet food, and many people feel that it is dangerous and may cause severe health problems. According to the U.S. Department of Health and Human Services, there are over ninety different documented symptoms and illnesses linked to aspartame. They include headaches, seizures, nausea, muscle spasms, weight gain, rashes, depression, fatigue, insomnia, hearing loss, heart palpitations, anxiety attacks, slurred speech, memory loss, joint pain, epilepsy, multiple sclerosis, Alzheimer's disease, and Parkinson's disease. Aspartame was discovered in 1965, but wasn't approved until 1981. Now you know why.

Besides diet soda, aspartame can be found in gum, breath mints, cereals, yogurt, frozen desserts, cocoa mixes, gelatin desserts, instant tea, and breakfast bars.

Maybe this stuff is okay in moderation, but I'm convinced that fake sweeteners give you the impression that more of everything is okay. Consequently, you could lose your ability to judge what a normal portion is. Or what moderation is.

As I learned more about health, people with better eating habits became attractive to me. I wanted to stop drinking the diet soda—but how, when I was so addicted?

I couldn't go cold turkey, so I traded in my convenience store "Big Gulps" for normal-sized cans of diet soda and sparkling water. I started with five cans and one bottle of sparkling water. I know five cans of diet

> Avoid any type of diet pill. Using diet pills to suppress your appetite sets you up for a number of nasty side effects such as high blood pressure, insomnia, irritability, dependence, and even death. Any weight you lose while taking them will come right back when you stop taking them.
>
> I'll say it again: people who eat breakfast usually feel less hungry throughout the day.

soda sounds like a lot, but it had a lot less caffeine and aspartame than the "Big Gulp." And I actually found the sparkling water refreshing! Each week I cut back one can of diet soda and added a bottle of sparkling water. Suddenly I didn't even like the taste of diet soda, but I couldn't get enough of the sparkling water!

I have always been a firm believer that YOU ARE WHAT YOU EAT. There is so much prepackaged, synthetic, preserved, dyed, "fake" food available that's full of ingredients you can't even pronounce.

Yes, I have to admit some of it does taste good. But what is it doing to the insides of our bodies? Do we really know? This stuff hasn't been around long enough for us to know the long-term effects. That's why I believe on sticking to "real" food. If it comes out of the ground or off a tree, then I'm going to opt for that.

I do not have anything with a sweetener in my house. And none of those little blue or pink packages. Real sugar, real butter—real food that's eaten in moderation. This way I know where it comes from, and I feel that I am always teaching myself (and my family) how to keep ourselves healthy so we can maintain and expand our level of fitness.

chapter five

Move It
and Use It

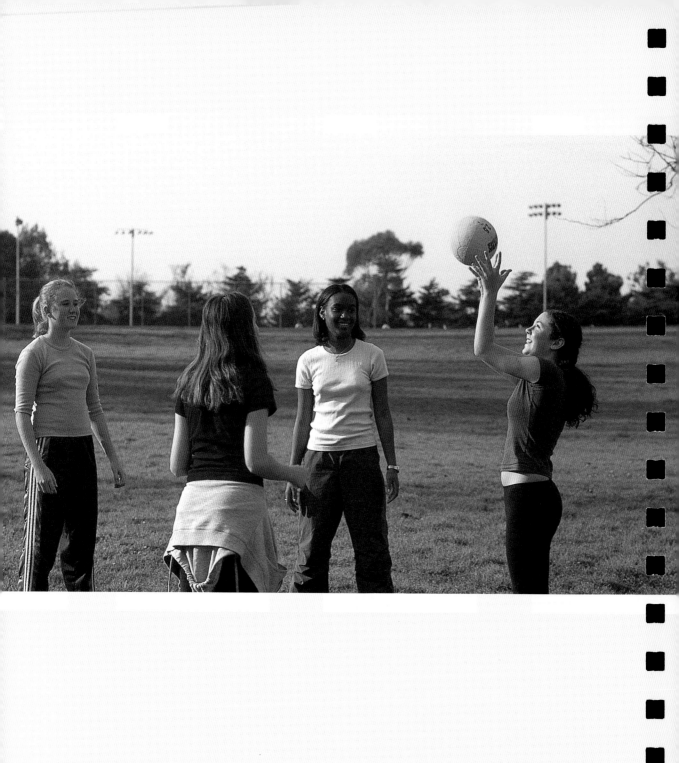

being the fitness consultant for *Today* for the last eight years has been a great experience for me. I get very creative for my segments, showing how fitness can be fun and never boring. I like to demonstrate exercises that you can do right in your home.

One of the funniest *Today* memories I have was when they were showing Christmas gift ideas in December 1999. Before I went on, the "Gadget Guru" was showing co-host Matt Lauer all kinds of unusual items for the home. On a big rug were two new fancy La-Z-Boy chairs and a small contraption. Once the segment started, the audience was told that weird-looking thing was a vacuum cleaner. Both Matt and the Gadget Guru relaxed into the chairs, holding remotes. The remotes were not for the television—they were for the vacuum cleaner!

I couldn't believe it. A household chore that creates a lot of exercise for anyone using it could now be done while sitting down.

After the demonstration, Matt and the Gadget Guru continued to discuss their feelings of comfort in these chairs as they described some of the options they offered. There was a holder for the remote and a holder for a snack and a drink. The big joke came when Matt said the only thing they lacked was a toilet. I think I will call it quits in the fitness industry if toilets are built into chairs. That will be the last straw!

time to get off our butts!

While the miracles of technology never cease to amaze me, there is a negative side to it all. For the majority of us, unless we take the time and make the effort to stay physical, technology literally sedates us. Since our bodies no longer get enough natural physical activity, our muscles are sluggish and sag at an earlier age than they did even twenty years ago. We need to get off our butts and make up for it in as many ways as possible by working out.

what is a workout?

One of my favorite definitions of what a workout is comes from George Allen, the former chairman of the President's Council for Physical Fitness and Sports: "A workout is 25 percent PERSPIRATION and 75 percent DETERMINATION."

Stated another way, it is one part physical exertion and three parts self-discipline. Doing it is easy once you get started—the trick is to keep doing it.

A workout makes you better today than yesterday. It strengthens your body, relaxes your mind, and toughens your spirit. Once you get started, and when you work out regularly, your problems seem to disappear and your confidence grows.

Working out is a personal triumph over laziness and procrastination. It is the badge of a winner, the mark of an organized, goal-oriented person who chooses to take charge of her destiny. A workout is a wise use of time and an investment in the most important thing in your life: yourself! It helps prepare you for life's challenges. Each time you complete a workout you've proven to yourself that you have "the right stuff." And you don't just feel better—you feel better about yourself!

A workout is a key that helps unlock the door to opportunity and success. Hidden within each of us is an extraordinary force. Physical and mental fitness are the triggers that can release it, helping us to achieve our goals.

your nearest gym is your home

If you've been living the life of a couch potato, where do you begin? (No one is expected to start running marathons overnight, if ever.) Whether you live in the city or the suburbs, you can begin in your own home with the basic exercise you get when you clean your house.

Nobody likes to "clean house"—but there is a way to turn household chores into a real workout. (I'm always looking for innovative ways to physically complicate every move I make. This allows me to get the most out of it.) So put on your sweats and sneakers, gather a bucket of cleaning supplies, turn on the radio, and really move! The trick is to go from one job to the next, without stopping, and *maximize your movements*. While you clean, dust, rearrange, and put away, focus on bending, stretching, and reaching as much as you possibly can, as you:

1. sweep the floors
2. scrub the kitchen and bathroom floors
3. clean out the refrigerator
4. scrub the cabinets
5. wash the windows
6. scrub the tub and shower
7. vacuum the house
8. make the beds
9. dust
10. wash the windows
11. clean out closets

These are just a few suggestions. Don't be afraid to be creative— there are no limitations. I'm sure, as you enter each room, you'll get more ideas. Also, when you watch television, why not do some sit-ups, push-ups, and leglifts. You can catch your favorite shows and do something good for your body at the same time.

creative fitness

Once you step out of the house, there are lots of ways to burn calories without even thinking about it. Here are some:

1. When you go to the mall, market, or the movies, park as far away as possible from your designated location. Make sure you are with someone and make it a fast walk. This will get your heart rate up and you will feel energized.

2. Take the stairs wherever and whenever. I always say to myself that elevators don't exist. There are times when you have to take them—but when you see those steps do not hesitate to use them.

3. Get up and manually change the channel on your television. I know this sounds silly, but you are moving your body, which means you are burning more calories. All these little activities add up.

4. Walk the dog. No excuses—no one is that busy. This is a great way to get a workout—there's that calorie burn again. It will make you feel better about yourself, and your dog will love you for it. For my three black Labs, it's the highlight of their day!

5. Invite some friends to rearrange your bedroom furniture. It's a great way to work up a really good sweat. Take a break and

then go on to someone else's house and rearrange their bedroom.

6. Spend Saturday mornings washing Mom's and Dad's cars. This is a great activity, not to mention fun—and you might even get paid! Best of all, if you put a time limit on yourself, it can turn into an aerobic workout.

7. Sign up for sports, whether they are offered by your school or by your local recreational department. This is a great way to meet new friends, try out a new sport, and work on getting in shape.

8. While you are waiting in line for a movie or waiting outside for a friend to pick you up, find a step, stair, or curb and walk up and down it. This is just like being in a step class without all the choreography. You will burn calories, and you will be surprised how quickly time flies!

9. Create a fitness contest with your family—or willing family members. You will be surprised how competitive everyone can get. Start with simple activities like how many push-ups and sit-ups everyone can do in 1 minute. Then move on to other activities, like who can walk around the block the quickest. How many pull-ups can everyone do?—you may have to go to a park for this one. Be creative, and before you know it, your entire family will achieve an improved fitness level.

10. Smile as much as possible! It exercises your face and in time will give you positive age lines.

suburban fitness

If you live in the suburbs, the following list is just the beginning of the numerous fun things you can do that will make your body healthier, stronger, and more fit:

1. Walk the dog . . . often!

2. Rake leaves, pull weeds, mow the lawn, plant flowers, make a rock garden—turn your yard into a visual masterpiece!

3. If you have a pool, take over maintaining it. You may want to let your parents handle the chemicals, but the brushing, vacuuming, and tile scrubbing really work your upper body. As an added bonus, you'll get a great tan—although make sure you use the appropriate sunblock to protect you from harmful ultraviolet rays.

4. Shovel snow.

5. Instead of being driven, or driving, ride your bike to get where you're going.

6. Shoot hoops in the driveway, at a friend's house, or at the local park.

7. Invite family members for a walk around the block after dinner.

8. Or how about a good old-fashioned game of kickball or kick-the-can?

9. Jump rope—alone or with your friends. Have contests to see who can last the longest.

10. Pool activities: don't float like a boat, dive for pennies, have relay races, organize a neighborhood water polo team.

11. Have a scavenger hunt with neighborhood friends—remember the team who finishes first with everything wins. This takes speed!

12. Wrestle with your parents, siblings, and friends.

13. If you baby-sit, which is usually a teen's first job, interact with the kids. Play tag, hide-and-seek, and any other active games. Not only will the kids fall fast asleep when put to bed, but you will become their favorite babysitter as well. It will also make the time go faster.

14. Unless it's unrealistic, get up earlier and walk to school with a friend. You'll feel refreshed instead of half-asleep for your first class.

15. Take a study break, put on your favorite music, and dance. Twenty minutes will pass in no time!

urban fitness

Living in a city does not have to exclude you from fitness. In fact, you have many more opportunities to walk places rather than drive. Including walking, here are some other ideas:

1. Get a group of friends together and walk the city blocks at a brisk pace. Being with friends will make the time fly and ensures safety.

2. Check out any local playgrounds for after-school sports activities. Make sure they're supervised and safe.

3. In every city across the country there is the YMCA, which offers numerous sports and exercise programs throughout the day.

4. Start jogging with a friend. When you come to traffic lights, simply jog in place until you can cross the street.

5. If you have a VCR, there are lots of inexpensive exercise tapes you can buy, including my own, which are listed in the appen-

dix, that will give you a terrific 20- to 45-minute workout. You may have to move some of the furniture around so that you have plenty of space to move. And no jazzy clothes are needed—just sweats or shorts and a T-shirt, and sneakers. Use the tape three times a week and I guarantee you'll like the way you look and feel after the first few weeks.

6. Invest in one piece of workout equipment, like a recumbent bike, that is collapsible and can be stored under a bed. (A recumbent bike, unlike a stationary bike, allows you to sit back and grip side handles as you pedal. It's great for working your stomach, hips, and thighs, and is easy on the back.) Five-pound free weights are good for daily upper body maintenance and are easily stored anywhere.

7. Go through your old magazines and cut out exercise routines from the fitness sections. Tape them to your mirror. (Some of the exercises may suggest that you use your 5-pound weights.)

8. Put a chin-up bar in the bathroom doorway and use it daily to build upper body strength.

9. Always take the stairs. In fact, if you live in an old brownstone, an elevator won't even exist.

10. In the city, shopping usually has to be done a couple of times a week. Volunteer to do it. Carrying bags while walking will give you an even greater workout.

11. City parks are great for bike riding, jogging, and Rollerblading.

Whether you're suburban or urban, my message to you is to move. Move your body whenever you can and maximize your movements.

As long as it's safe, walk or ride your bike instead of getting a ride. Put that box of tissues at the opposite end of your nightstand so that you'll have to stretch your muscles and reach. When the phone rings—why not run to the one farthest away from you to get that extra bit of exercise? You might be in the kitchen, but why not use the upstairs bathroom instead of the powder room?

The point is, move it and use it whenever you can. Let your body fully operate as the wonderful machine that it is. It has the capacity to be a real workhorse and it's counting on you to put it to use. Don't let technology ruin it. Remember, you're in control of your body.

chapter six

The Five-Minute Workout

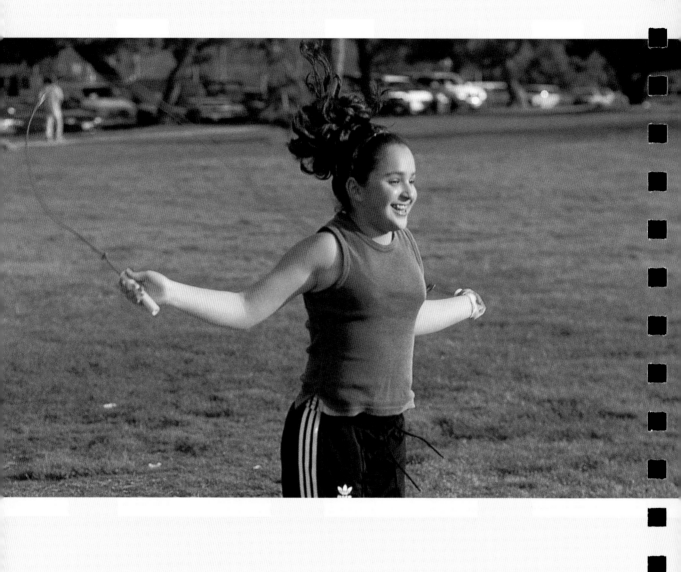

Wake up and tighten up! Think of the following 5 minutes as your daily body booster.

This workout can be done when you get up in the morning, in your bedroom, before you shower. You don't need to change out of your pj's, and you don't need any shoes. But if you prefer, a pair of comfortable sweatpants and a T-shirt will do the trick.

This workout will get the blood flowing, wake up your muscles, and get you out of your sleep groove. It's a great way to jump-start your day as you tone your arms, abs, outer thighs, and butt.

stand and reach

Stand up straight and reach to the ceiling with both arms. Hold this stretch and continue to reach even higher.

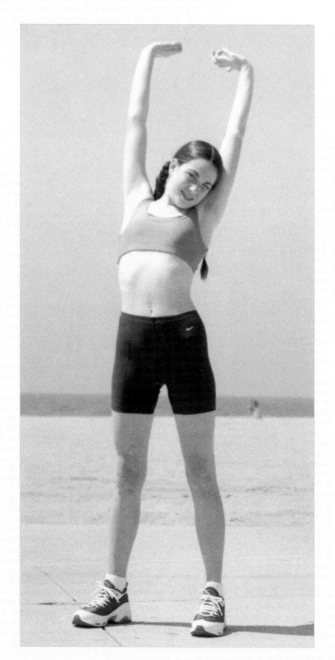

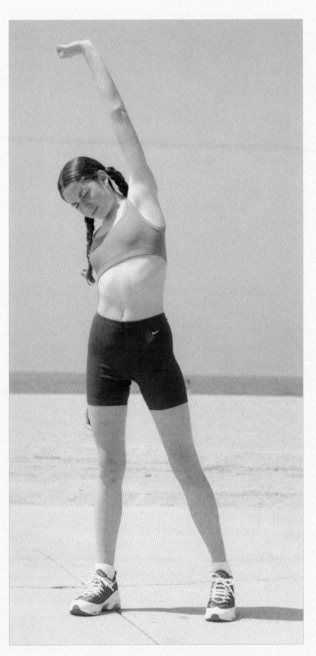

Reach with one arm up,
hand above your head, and
feel the stretch all the way
down your sides.
Switch arms.

shoulder rolls

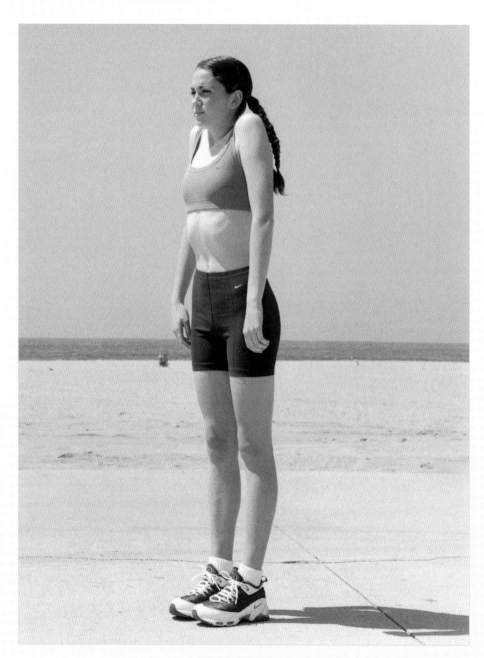

Roll your shoulders up, back, and down four to five times.

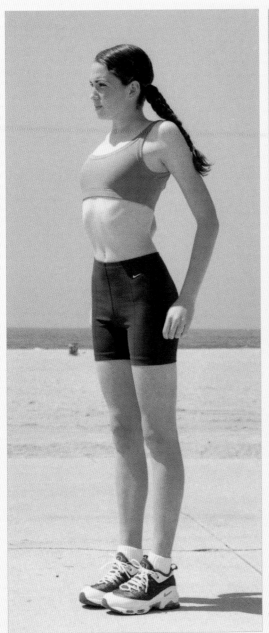 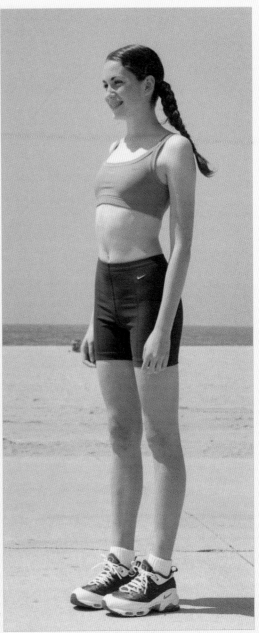

shoulders up and stretch

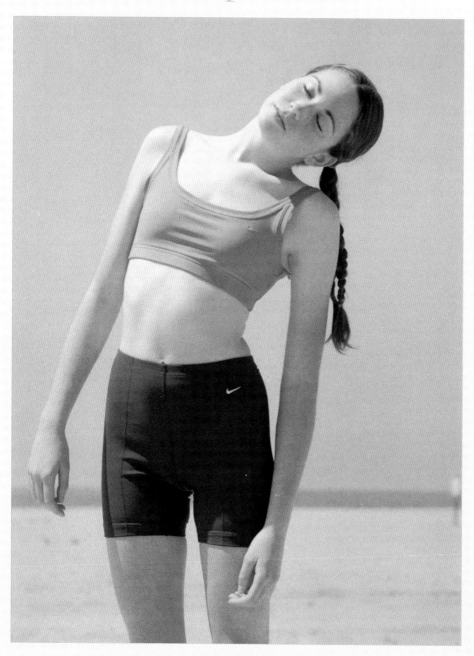

With your shoulders down, tilt your head to one side, bringing one ear toward your shoulder. Hold. Now repeat on the other side and hold it. (On either side, do not allow your shoulder to come up and touch your ear.)

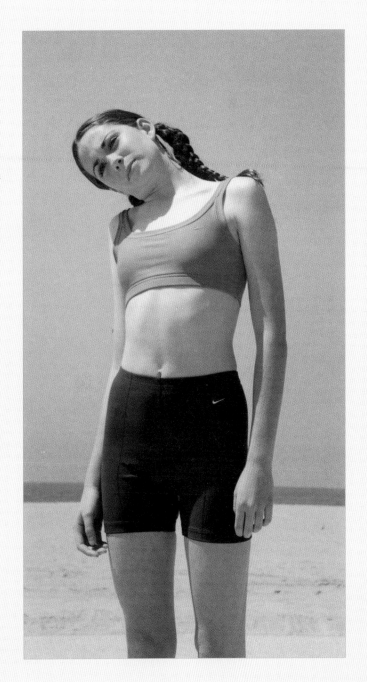

plié

Step out so that your feet are a little more than shoulder width apart. Keep your knees slightly bent. Your back is straight and your abs are pulled in tight. As you lower yourself down, your knees should follow out in a line directly over your toes. Your toes should point at the 10 and 2 o'clock positions.

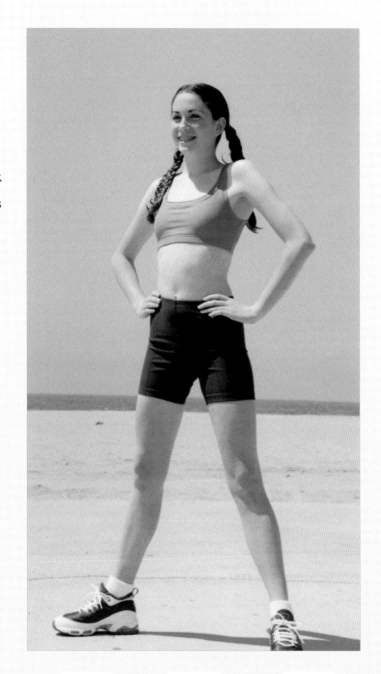

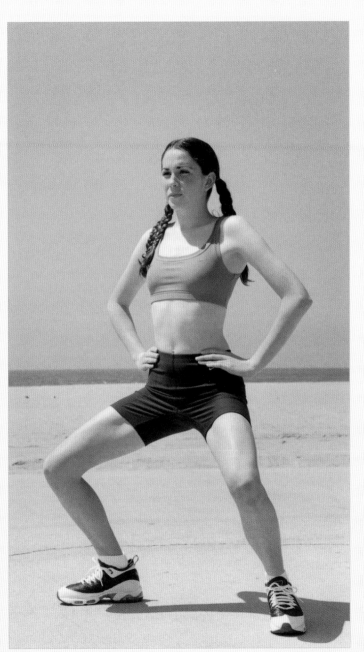

Go down so that your hips are parallel to your knees and then come back up. Keep your knees slightly bent at the top. Do not hold or pause at the top or bottom of your plié. Squeeze your butt together as tight as you can as you come up. Do 30 repetitions with an upbeat tempo. You will feel this in the front of your thighs and in your butt.

knee up and reach

Standing tall, bring one knee up toward your chest and reach both arms up in the air. Repeat with the other knee. Do 30 repetitions.

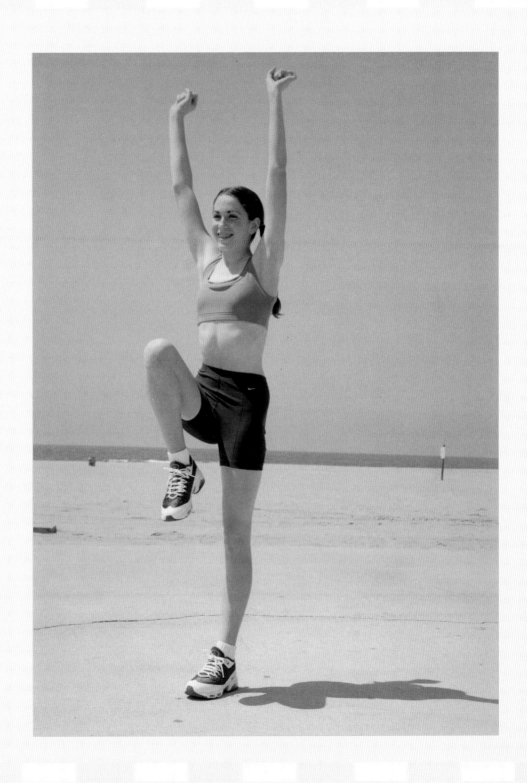

triceps dip

Sit on the edge of a desk chair or on the edge of the tub in your bathroom. Grab the edge with your hands. With your knees bent, slide your butt off the seat. Bending at your elbows, dip your butt down toward the ground in front of the chair or tub. Straighten your arms and raise yourself back up. *Do not lock your elbows.* Keep your body close to the chair or tub—don't lean back. Begin with 8 repetitions, working up to 15 at a time.

This exercise tones and tightens the backs of your upper arms. This is the area you want to look hot if you are wearing tank, tube, or halter tops! Pull your desk chair out and sit on the edge of it, or sit on the edge of the tub. With knees bent, slide your butt off the seat. Dip down, bending at your elbows until your elbows are parallel to your shoulders. Come back up. *Do not lock your elbows.* Begin with 8 repetitions and build up so that you can do 15 in a row. This exercise is good for your triceps, which run along the backs of your arms.

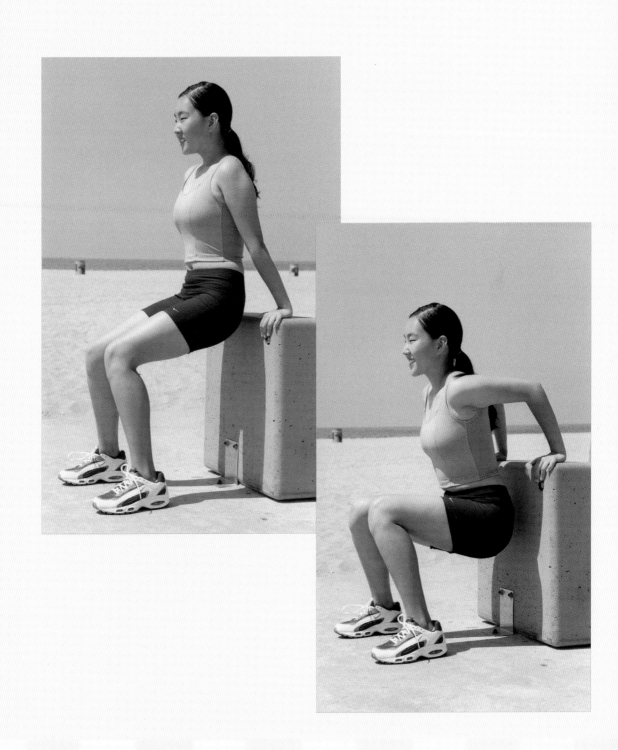

leglift series

The combination of these two leg exercises will shape and tone the outsides of your thighs like never before. Squeeze your butt as tight as you can as you go through the repetitions. Keep your abs pulled in and flex your foot.

On the floor, lie on your side. Prop yourself up on your elbow. Keep your body straight. Pull your knees in toward your chest. Lift the top leg up and down. Keep your knee facing forward throughout the lift. This will help you isolate your outer thigh. Do 30 repetitions.

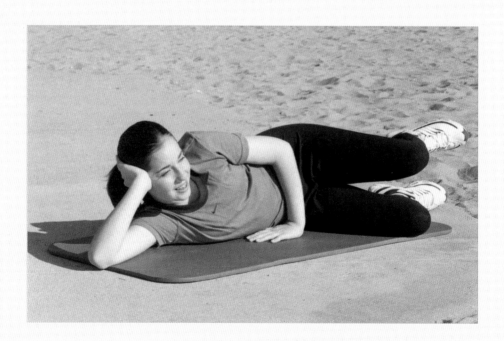

Remain in the same position, but instead of lifting the leg straight up, make small circles with the knee. Do 15 in one direction and then switch sides. Repeat the first leg exercise for 30 and then the circles for 15.

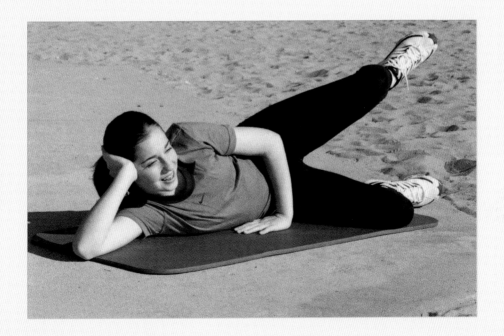

stretch it all out

Roll onto your back and pull both knees into a stretch. This stretch will feel so good after the burn of the leglifts. You should feel relief in your butt and lower back. While hugging your knees into your chest you will also feel a stretch in your upper back. Take a few deep breaths to relax into the stretch. Remember, stretching is supposed to feel good, so never pulse or pull it. Just hold it and breathe.

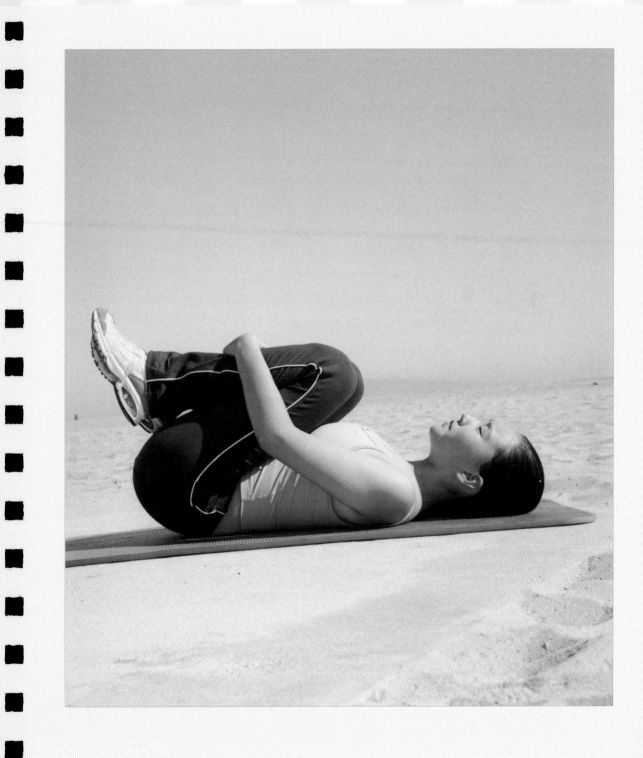

absolutely abs

Here are three ab workouts to get a trimmer tummy. These moves strengthen the torso and lower back muscles. You will also improve your balance and posture.

ab crunch

Lie on your back and bring your knees up toward your chest. Place your hands behind your head, exhale, inhale, and lift up toward your thighs. Breathe out as you come up. Inhale when you are returning to the starting position. Do 30 repetitions. This will help you isolate your abdominal muscles and flatten your belly.

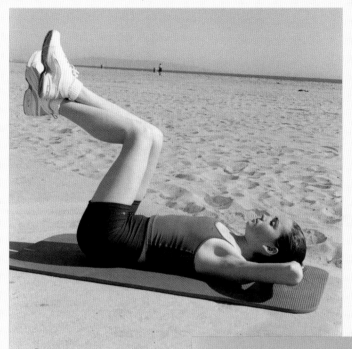

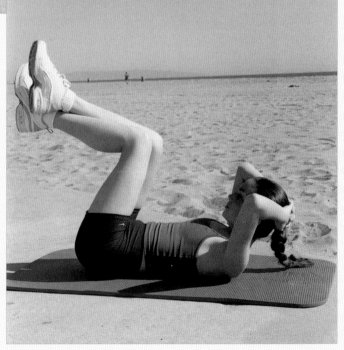

knee in crunch

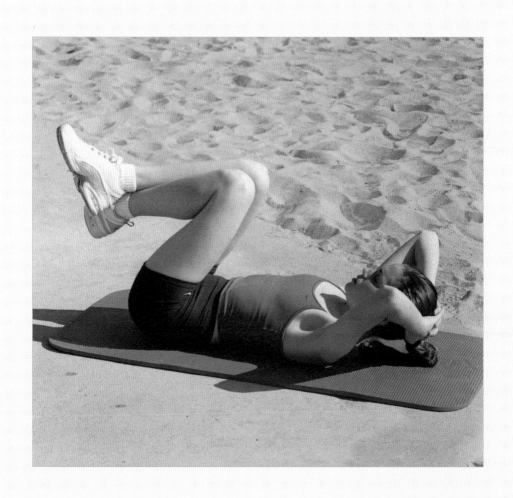

Stay in the same position as the ab crunch. As you crunch, pull your knees in toward your chest as you lift up toward your thighs. You will feel this burn up and down your abs. Keep your chin off your chest and continue with the same breathing technique. Do 30 repetitions.

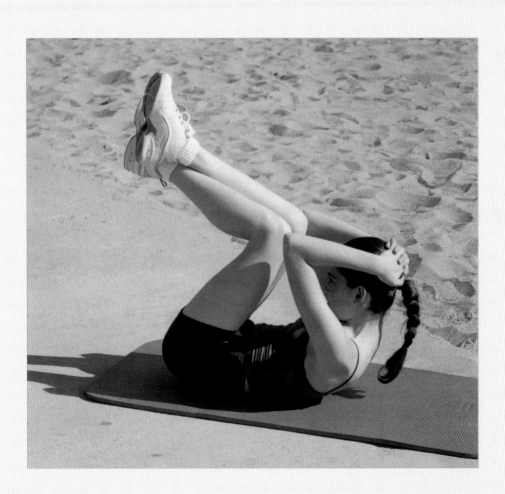

oblique crunch

This is the best crunch to cinch your waistline. The oblique muscle wraps around you like a corset and will pull in your middle section.

Keep the same position as the ab crunch. Keeping your feet and knees up, hands behind your head, lift and reach one elbow toward the opposite knee. Focus on something over your knee and reach up to it instead of twisting over. Do 30 repetitions on each side.

For quicker results, go back to the first ab exercise and repeat the whole series. *You will need a few extra minutes, but I think you will like the results.*

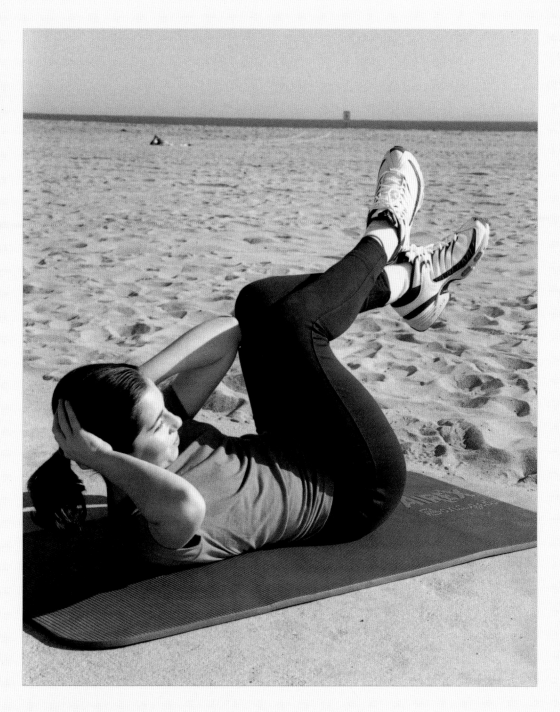

backside toner

This exercise is great for your lower body. You will see shape and tone and a distinct separation between the butt and the backs of the legs. (Well-conditioned legs look sexy!) Extra calories will be burned, and there will be a gradual decrease in overall body fat.

To start, lie on your back with one heel resting on the seat of a chair. Your upper body should remain flat on the floor. The other leg extends straight up in the air.

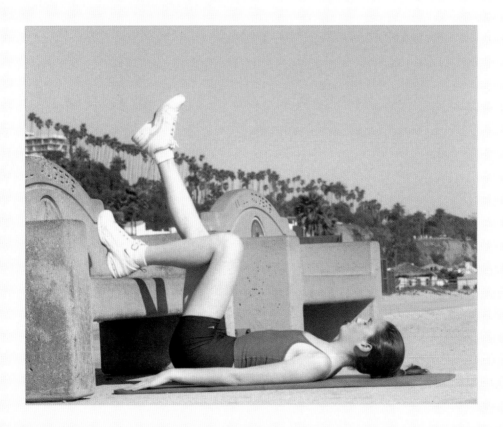

Keep the straight leg stationary. Your bent knee should make a right angle so that your hip is directly under your knee. Play around with the position so that you can really isolate the back of your leg.

Press your heel into the chair, squeeze your butt muscle, and lift your body without lifting your shoulder blades. Slowly lower back down. Do 15 repetitions and then repeat with the other leg.

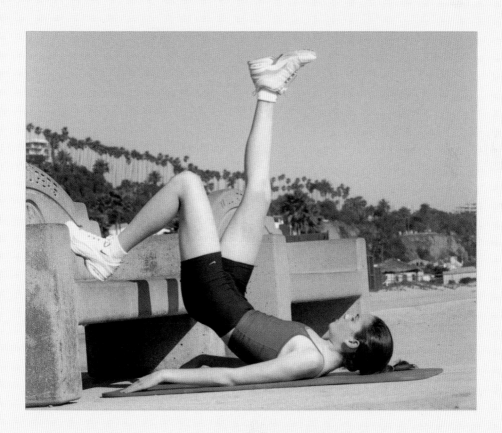

stand and reach

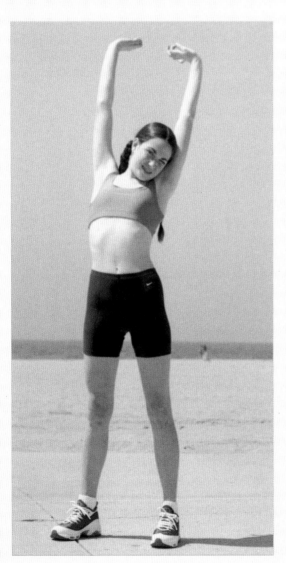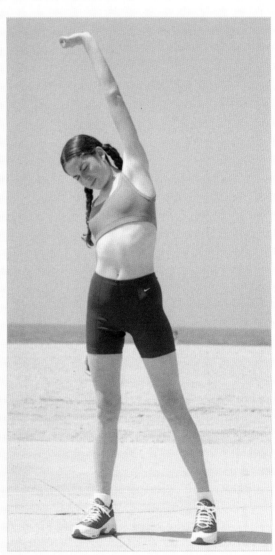

Stand and repeat the beginning stretches. Now it's off to the shower. You should feel awake and alive. Congratulations! You have done something great for your body today.

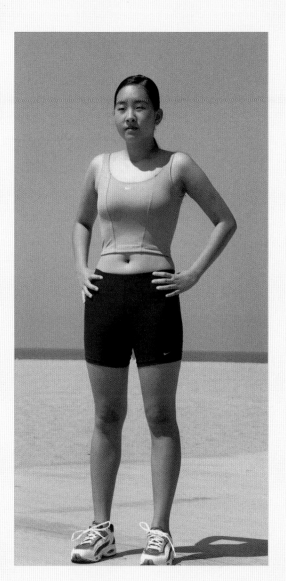

If you can't do all of the repetitions that I have recommended, don't worry. Start out with as many as you can do and build up from there. If this workout takes you more than 5 minutes, then that is a goal you can shoot for. See if you can shave off a little bit of time each time you do this routine. You will be amazed at how quickly your body responds if you are consistent, doing this workout every day. It is fun and easy— yet challenging.

chapter seven

The Twenty-Minute Workout

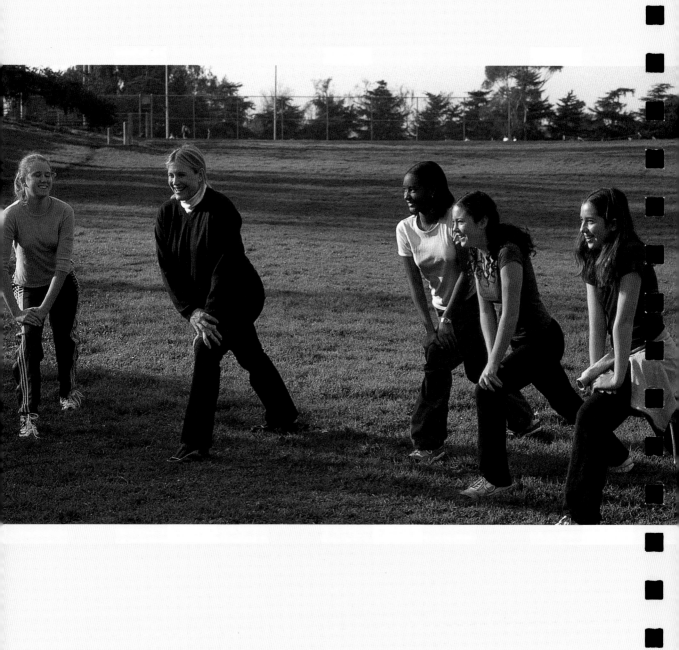

this is an ultrafun workout that you can do by yourself or with your best friend. This workout will get you fit. It's got everything in it! Cardio, strength training, toning, shaping, and stretching. You will achieve awesome arms, abs, butt, and legs if you do this on a regular basis. This means at least three times a week. So grab a buddy, or if she's off at the mall, start sweating on your own. All you need is the equipment shown below, some comfy sweats or workout tights, a T-shirt, and a good pair of cross-trainer shoes. If you don't have cross-trainers, running or aerobic shoes are fine. And don't forget your breasts—they need the extra support you get from a good sports bra.

You may laugh, but some teens and women have a hard time exercising because of their large breasts. The numerous inadequate sports bras don't help, nor does the difficulty in finding the right size.

My client Drew Barrymore started training with me while she was preparing for the movie *Charlie's Angels* because she needed to be in better than great shape. We started with fast walking and some weight training. I then wanted to move her on to running, jump rope, and some other high-impact exercise—but the look on her face told me this was not going to happen. Embarrassed, she admitted to me that she couldn't do those activities because they hurt her chest—specifically her breasts.

I had the perfect solution for her: the Enell bra. This is a tight bra vest with eye-hook fastenings. Tears came to her eyes when she got back on the treadmill and started running. She was elated. Without feeling any pain, she was now able to run. You must always protect your body from head to toe in order to avoid injuries. To obtain an Enell sports bra, refer to the Appendix at the end of the book.

the equipment used in the twenty-minute workout

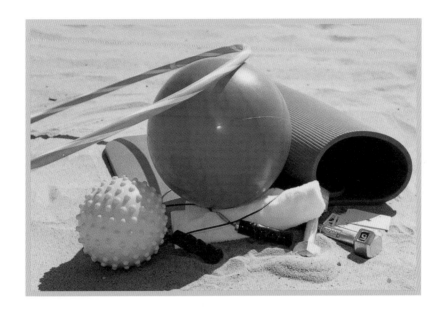

Ball *(This is a large ball found in sports stores. See the Appendix for more information.)*

Jump Rope

Towel

Weights

Hula Hoop

Mat

10 Playing Cards

Let's Begin!

warming up

Warming up your body is really important before you begin to exercise. It gets your body ready. You should feel your heart rate kick up and your breathing should increase—it's the same feeling you get when you see that guy you've been eyeing.

You can do any one of the three warm-ups that are shown or you can do all three. You only need to warm up for 5 minutes, followed by some stretching. When you stretch, make sure you hold it until you feel gentle tension. Breathe into the stretch. Don't push or bounce. Hold each position for 30 to 60 seconds.

1.

FAST WALKING: walk around the block or around your house.

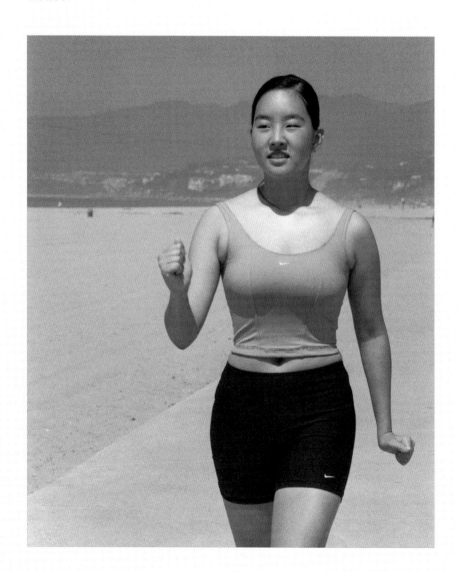

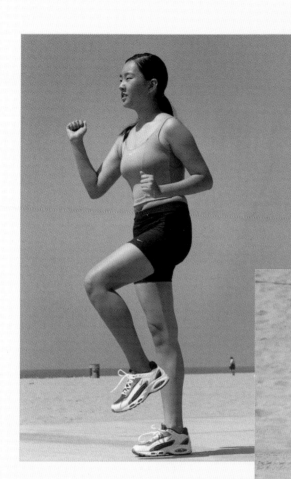

MARCHING IN PLACE: march in place until you feel revved up.

CLIMBING STAIRS:
walk up and down a
few flights of stairs to get
warmed up.

2. quadriceps stretch

Stand with your feet together. Pull your ankle up from behind toward your hip. Hold the stretch. Make sure to keep your knees together and do not lean forward. Press down toward the ground with the bent knee and feel your quadriceps muscle lengthen. Hold as long as you can, and then switch sides.

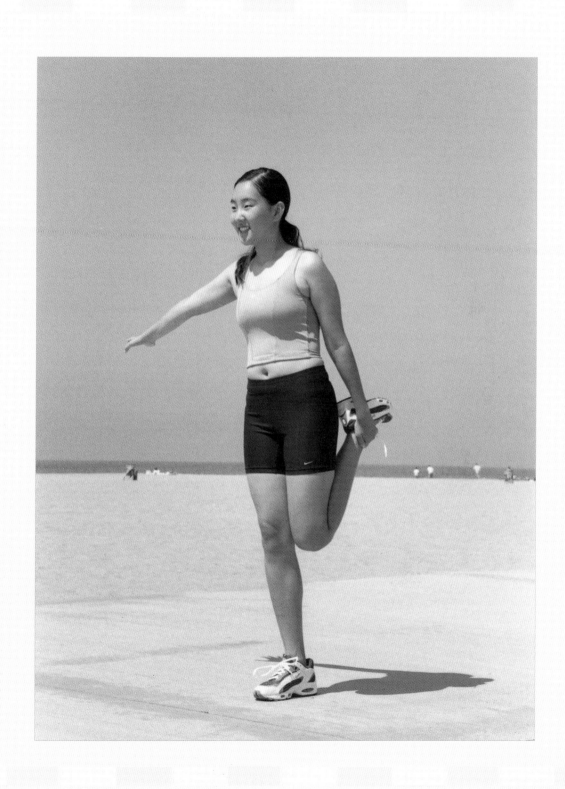

3. standing hamstring stretch

Flex your body forward at your hips. Bend one knee and extend your other leg straight out in front of you. Place your hands on your bent knee for balance. Flex the foot of your straight leg and feel the stretch in the back of your leg. Hold for as long as you can. To increase the stretch, lean forward as you breathe into the stretch and feel your hamstring lengthen. *Never bounce these stretches, always hold.* Switch your legs and repeat.

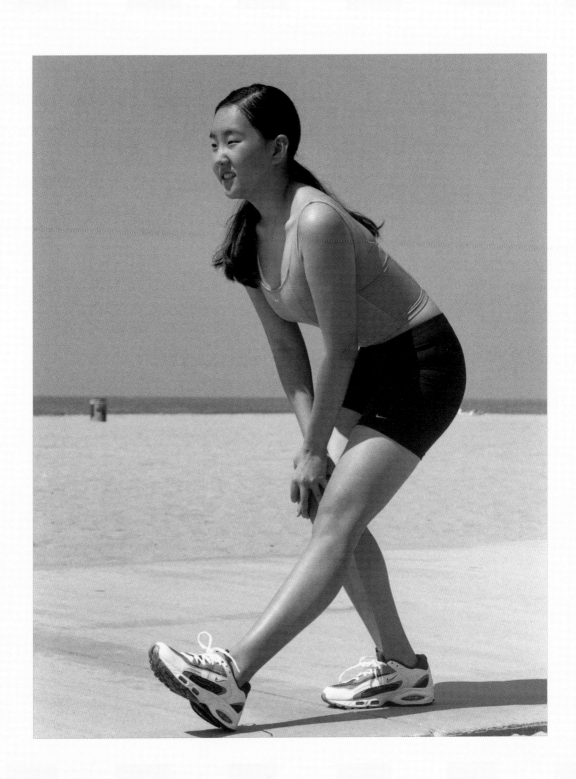

4. calf stretch

Standing upright, step back with a straight leg. Press heel down until you feel the stretch in your straight leg. By keeping your heel down, you are stretching from your Achilles tendon up through your calf. Hold this position for as long as you can, and then switch your legs.

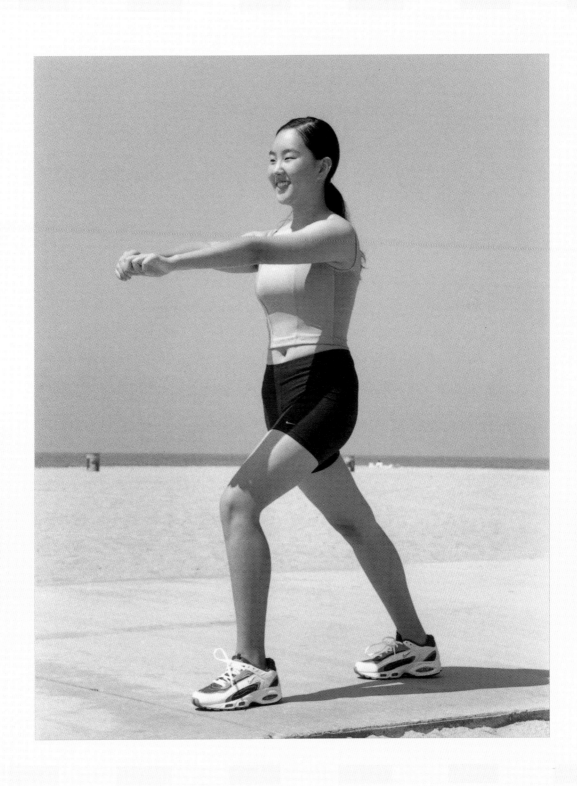

cardio one—the fat blaster

If you are with a partner, one of you will jump rope, and one of you will use the hula hoop. Jump or hula for 2 minutes. Then switch with your partner and go for another 2 minutes.

If you're working out alone, jump rope for 2 minutes and then use the hula hoop for 2 minutes.

The hula hoop is a great piece of equipment to use to whittle and shape your waistline. It also helps to improve coordination. Put the hoop on the floor and stand in the middle. Bring the hoop up to your waist. Throw the hoop to one side of your hips and begin moving back and forth as if you're dancing, shifting your hips from side to side. Don't give up—you'll get the hang of it soon.

You are now 4 minutes into your workout. This does not include your 5-minute warm-up.

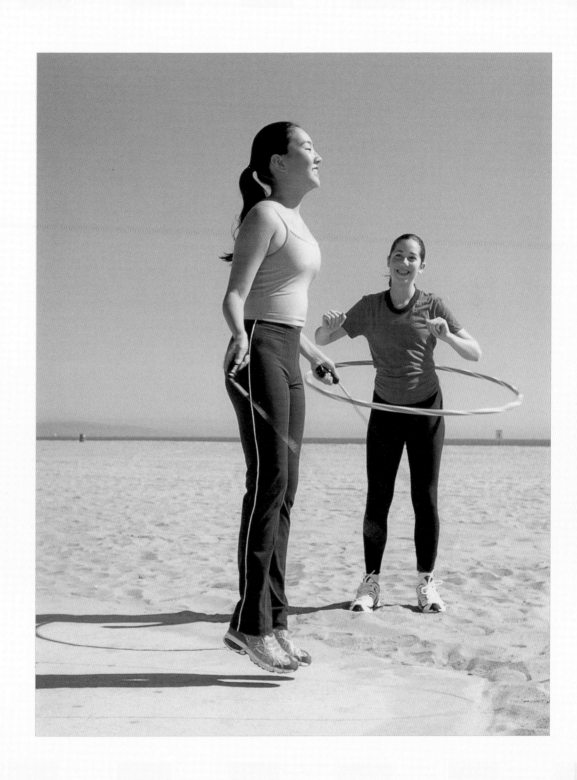

first strength workout

partner workout

super stance

The super stance will improve your balance and tone your legs. This exercise should be done on a soft surface.

Stand facing your partner. Place your feet shoulder width apart. Hold your partner's forearms just above her wrists. Put one foot on your partner's thigh right above the knee. Leading with your right foot, step up onto your partner's thighs. Slowly lean back and straighten out your body. Holding this pose, count to 60 or hold as long as you can. Now it's her turn.

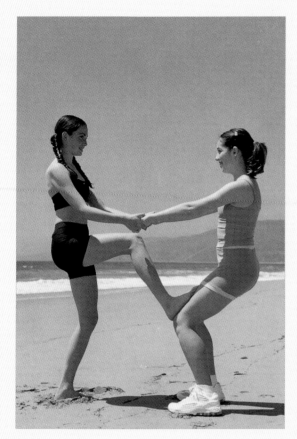

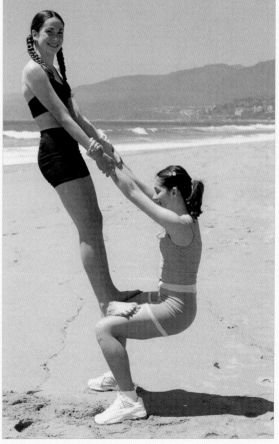

wall sit

The wall sit will improve the tone in your legs.

Lean up against a sturdy wall and slide back down until your hips are at the same level as your knees. Your feet should extend far enough that your knees are directly over your ankles. Remain in this position for the count of 60.

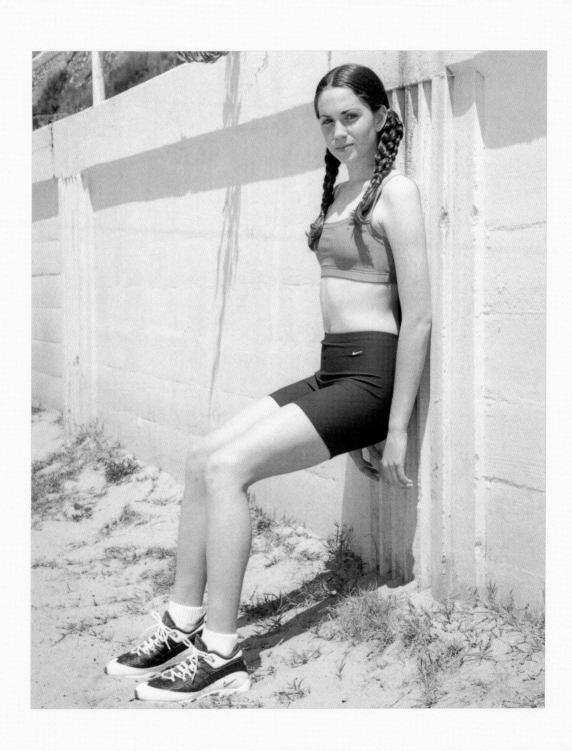

wall push-ups

This exercise is great for toning your chest and shoulders. It also improves your upper body strength.

Stand about 2 to 3 feet away from the wall. Place your hands against the wall so they're somewhat wider than shoulder width. Lower yourself toward the wall while bending your elbows. Turn your head to one side. If you do not feel this in your shoulders and your chest, then you are standing too close to the wall. Make sure you breathe out as you push away from the wall. Do 20 repetitions.

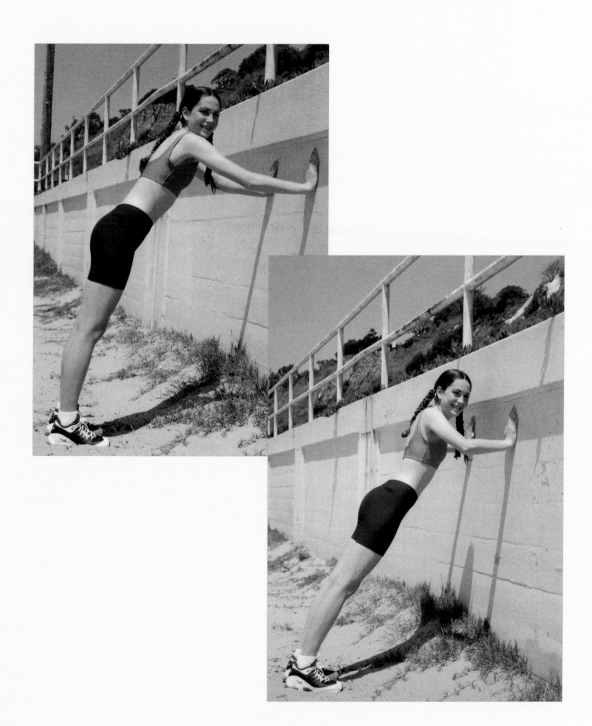

playing cards

The ultimate way to lift your butt and get rock-hard legs. You will definitely feel this and love the way it works. All you do is lunge forward and backward as you pick up playing cards. Sounds easy? Do it correctly and you'll really feel it working on your butt and legs.

Place 10 cards down in a pile in front of you. Take a big step back (both feet). Then:

- Lunge forward with your right leg toward the cards. Your right foot should land with its instep right next to the cards. When you land, your right knee is directly over your ankle. Your back left knee should be bent.

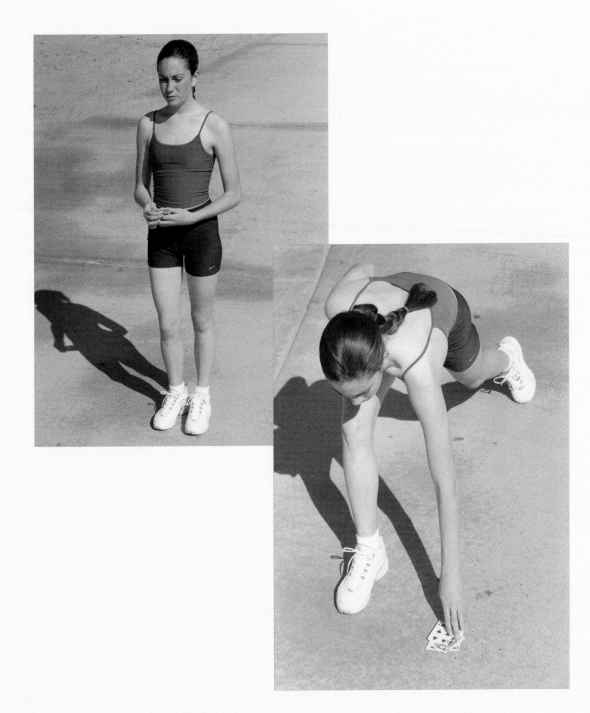

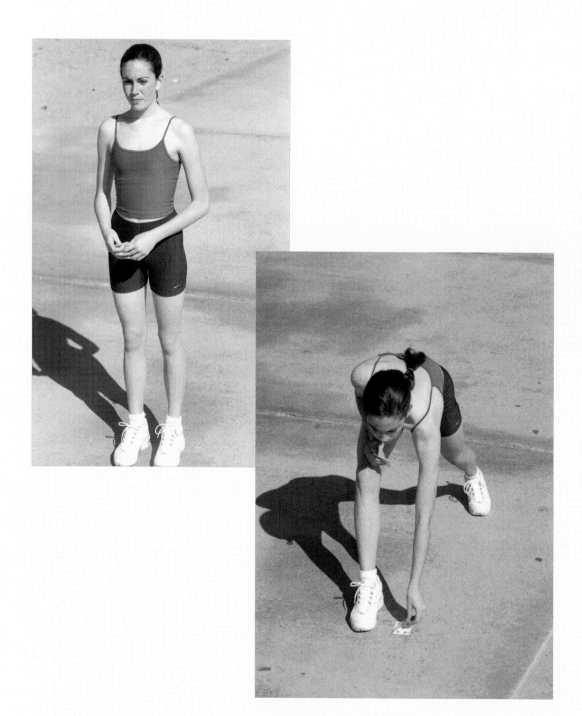

- Reach down with your left hand and pick up 1 card. Make sure that you lower your entire body to pick up the card.
- With your right leg, push back to the beginning position. Put the card in your right hand.
- Now lunge backward with your right leg. Lower your entire body and place the card at the instep of your left foot. Bring your right leg forward to the beginning position.
- You've just completed 1 repetition. Continue until you've used all 10 cards.
- Repeat, lunging forward and backward with the left leg.

(Helpful hint for lunging: step forward with one leg. Keep your chest up and back straight. Lower your body by bending at the knees. Your front knee should be directly over your ankle. Go down as far as you can without the back knee touching the ground. Tighten your butt as you push back to the starting position. If you find yourself off balance, your stride is too far apart. This can be corrected by bringing your legs closer together.)

second cardio workout

Return to the first cardio workout. Repeat workout with the jump rope and hula hoop. Remember, whether alone or with a partner, you'll be alternating 2 minutes with the hula hoop and 2 minutes with the jump rope.

second strength workout
partner workout

power arms

This exercise is great for toning your arms. Definition and tightness will develop—something we all want, especially when we are wearing sleeveless tops!

Stand with your partner directly in front of you. Her arms should be at her sides. Place your arms directly over hers. Your knees should be slightly bent. You will be acting like a weight machine. Have your partner lift her arms to shoulder level. Applying pressure, give her as much resistance as she needs. You can tell if you are not giving her enough pressure when she can lift and lower her arms with ease. If she can't move her arms at all, you are applying too much pressure. The goal is for her to have to work, but not struggle to lift her arms. Do 15 repetitions.

Stay in the same position, but this time have her begin with her arms straight out at shoulder level. Place your arms on top of hers. Now try to push

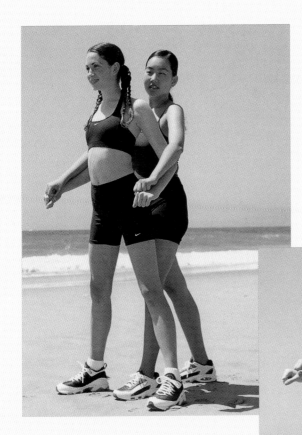

her arms down while she tries to push them up. Remember, you are only the weight machine, so if she is not getting anywhere, then you are pressing down too hard. Do 15 repetitions. Switch positions so that she is the weight machine.

partner push-ups

Place yourself in the push-up position on a mat. Your knees should be bent, and your hands shoulder width apart. Keep your back straight. Imagine that your torso is a board. Look down at the mat. Keep your abs pulled in tight and do not lock your elbows. Your partner will now straddle your body and squat down to place her hand gently on your upper back. Between the shoulder blades is best. As you move down toward the mat, inhale. Bring yourself as close to the mat as possible, without sagging in the middle of your torso. As you push up, exhale. Hold the position as your partner applies resistance by pressing down on your back. Start with 10 repetitions and then switch with your partner. As you get stronger, you may want to try 15 to 20 repetitions. If you can't do them with the resistance from your partner, then you both should do the push-ups on your own until you improve your strength.

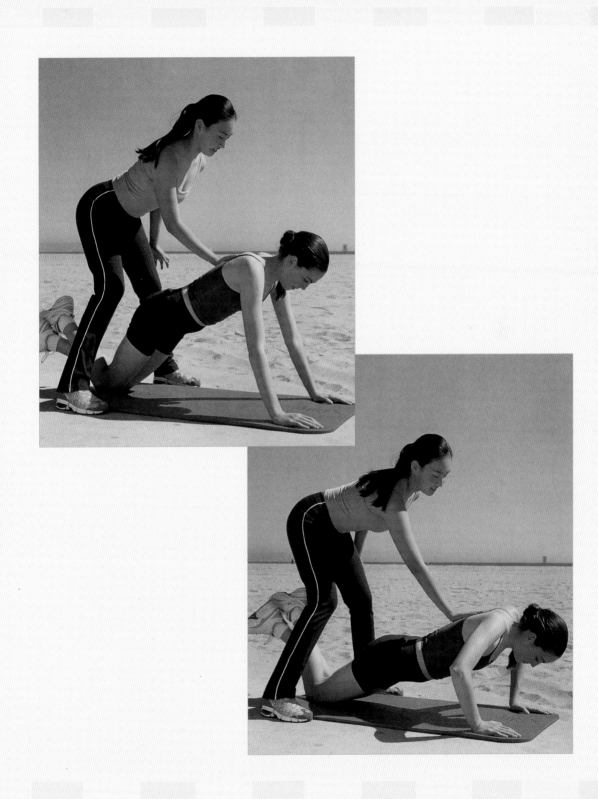

Use 5-pound weights for these upper body exercises.

Do 10 to 15 repetitions of each one of these exercises, depending on how strong you are. Do one exercise after another with no rest in between. To get started, get your body into a tabletop position. Slightly bend your knees and flex forward at your waist. Your back should be as straight as possible.

rear fly

Hold the weights in your hands, with your arms hanging straight down. Lift your arms so that they are even with your shoulders as you squeeze your shoulder blades together. The muscles you are using are the rear deltoids (located at the back of each shoulder). This is the area I call the "bra strap area." The rear fly is a very good exercise to keep it tight and toned.

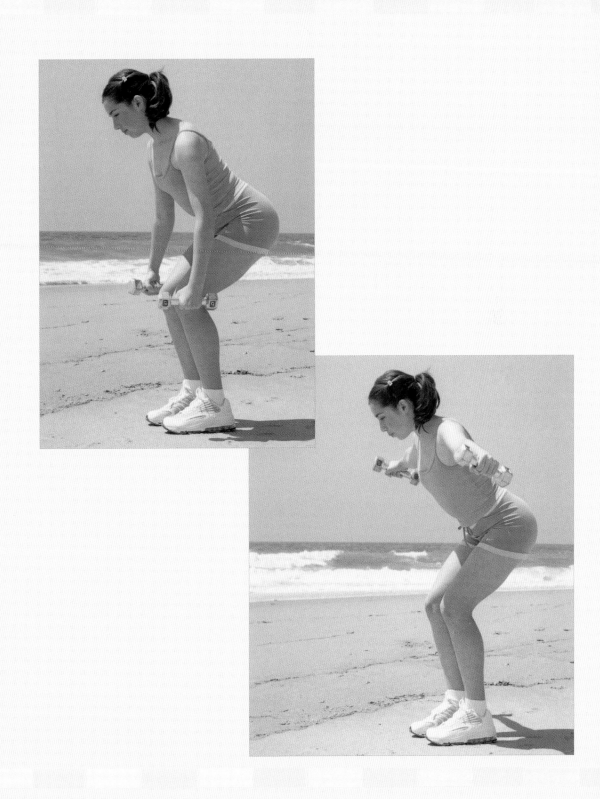

triceps
extension

Stay in the same body position as for the rear fly, only now you will be working your triceps, the backs of your arms—an area we all want tightened, toned, and defined. After you complete the last rear fly, bring your elbows up so that they hug the side of your body next to your rib cage. Keeping elbows in this position, extend both arms back until they are straight. Do not move your elbows. This will help isolate your triceps. As you extend back, exhale. Keep your abs tight, and squeeze the backs of your arms.

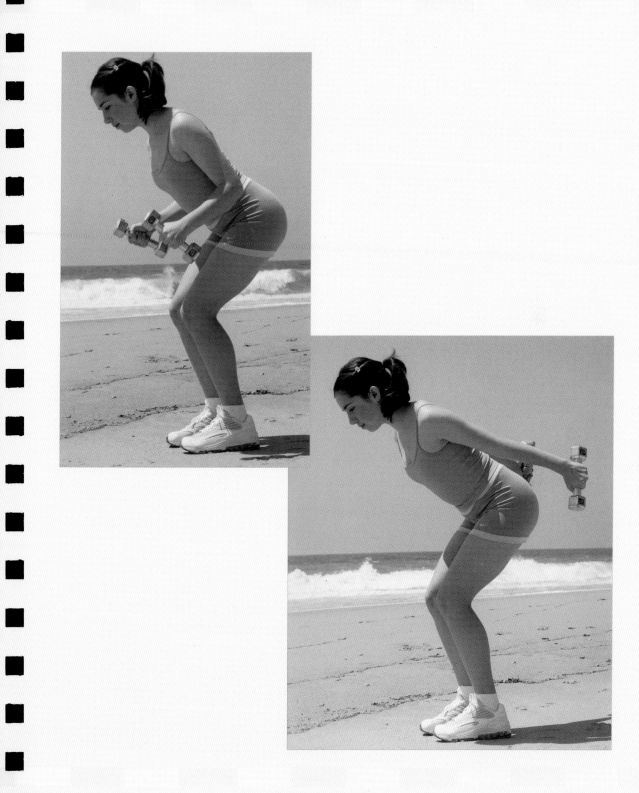

overhead
press

Standing upright, bring the weights to your shoulders, palms facing out. Press up until your arms are almost straight, but do not lock your elbows. Exhale as you press up and inhale as you bring your arms down. This is another great shoulder exercise that tones, strengthens, and defines.

Remember, with each of these exercises, focus on your breathing. An easy way to remember to do this is to exhale on the effort. So if you are pushing up, then breathe out. Inhale on the relaxation phase of the exercise.

These are the last two exercises in the workout. They must be done solo. If you are working with a partner you can both do them at the same time.

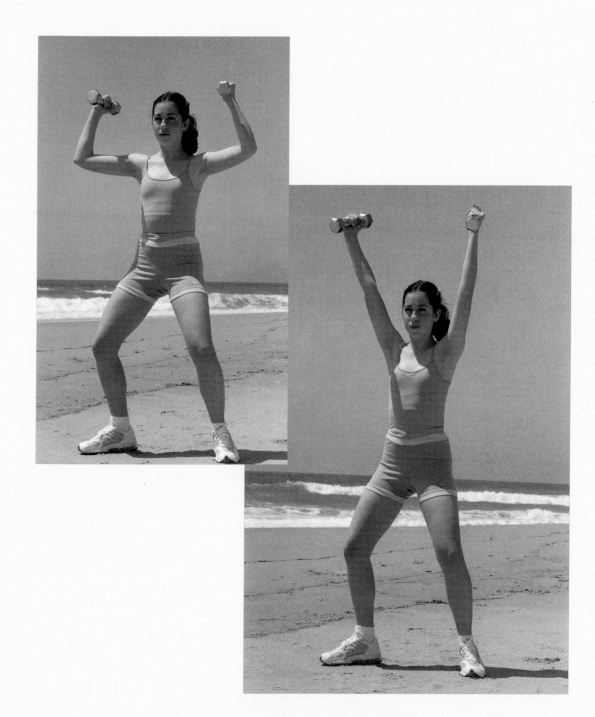

inner thigh
squeeze

You will need a medium-sized ball for this one. I have used a little beach ball, a basketball, a volleyball, or you can get an exercise ball at your local sporting goods store.

Lie on your back with your knees bent and your feet flat on the ground. Place the ball between your knees and hold it there. Create some light tension with your inner thighs. Your hands can rest on the ground next to you. To start, squeeze the ball as if you are going to pop it. Release slightly, still holding the contraction. Keep some gentle tension there. Then repeat. The contractions are not fast. Exhale each time you squeeze the ball. Really feel the isolation in your inner thighs. This is a great exercise to tighten your thighs and give your legs a great shape. Do 25 repetitions.

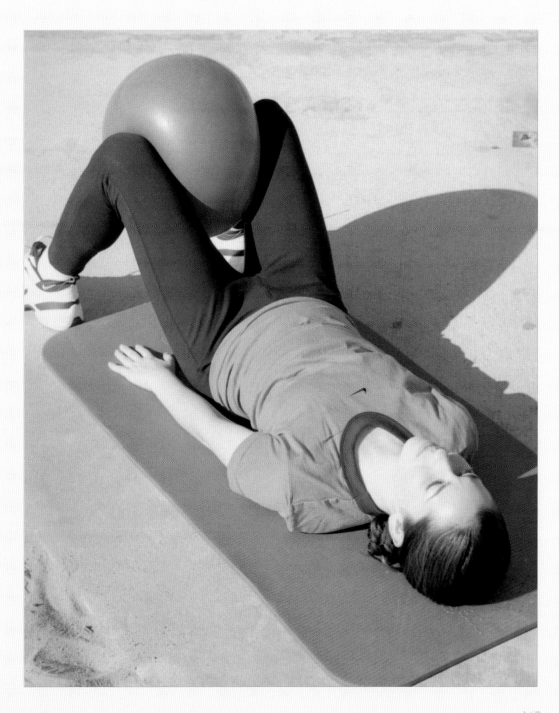

abdominal
crunch

If you want to work toward a toned belly, this is the exercise you had better memorize. Along with proper diet and aerobic exercise, doing these crunches will give tone and shape to your abs.

Stay on your back. Hands are behind your head, knees are bent, and feet are flat on the ground. Lift your upper body until your

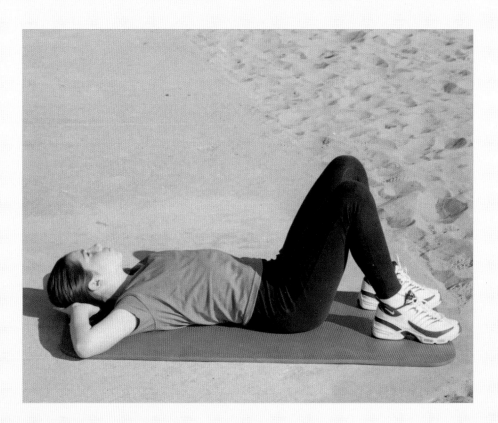

shoulder blades come off the ground. (Do not pull your chin into your chest. Look up and over your knees.) Exhale as you come up. Inhale as you go down. Blowing all your breath out as you come up teaches you how to flatten your belly. Repeat 25 times.

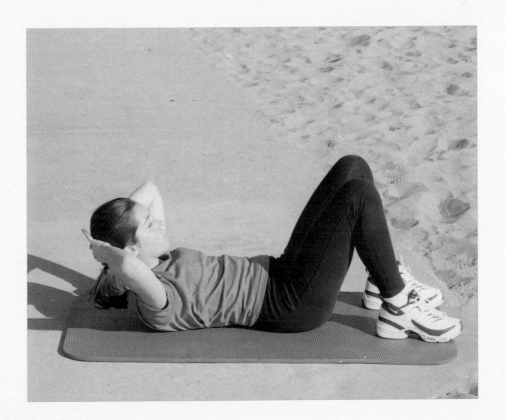

cool down

hamstring stretch

Lie on your back and take a towel and wrap it around the instep of your foot or calf, depending how flexible you are. Holding the ends of the towel in both hands, pull your leg in gently toward your chest. You will feel this stretch in the back of your leg. Hold for at least 1 minute. As you feel your flexibility improve, keep pulling the towel in tighter toward your chest. Repeat on your other leg

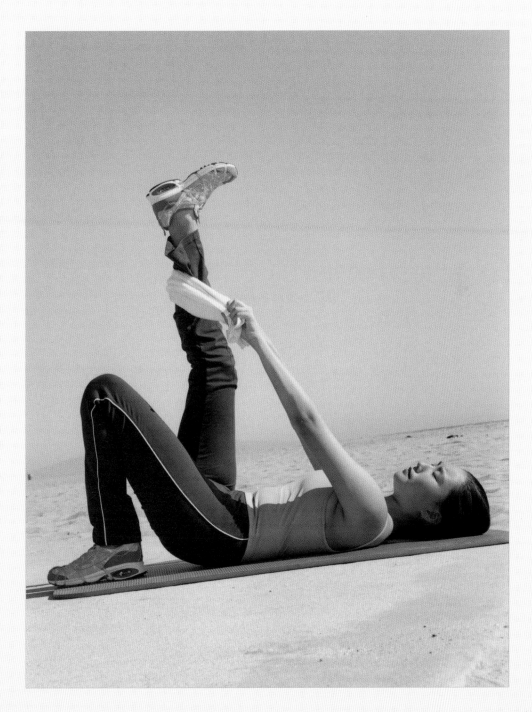

quadriceps
stretch

Flip over onto your belly. Hold your ankle or your shin with one hand. Gently pull your thigh off the mat and feel the stretch in the front of your thigh. Hold for at least 1 minute.

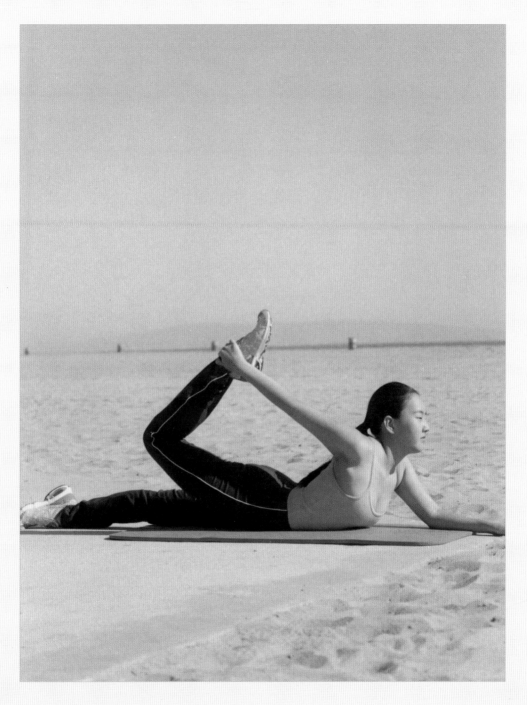

total body lengthening

Lie on your back. Reach your arms overhead and point your toes. Now imagine your entire body longer, and hold it. Continue to stretch in that fashion, imagining that you are getting longer. Finish with some deep breathing.

A note about lengthening: you often hear about exercises that lengthen your muscles, when in truth this is impossible. Your muscles don't work that way. You can definitely improve your flexibility, which may make you feel as if you have longer muscles—but it is just a feeling. The best thing to do is to use these workouts consistently and to continue to challenge yourself from now on. You will thank yourself in the years to come.

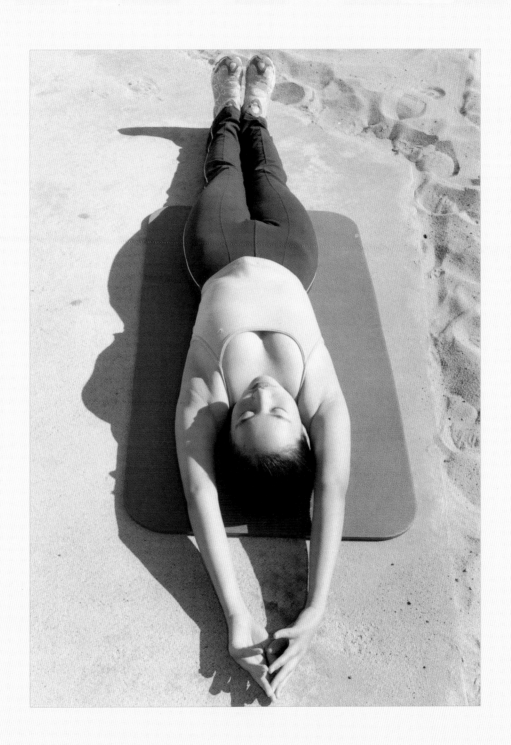

From the beginner to the athlete, these two workouts are for everyone. If you're just beginning and find yourself struggling with the repetitions, do as many as you can—but sometimes we all have to grit our teeth and push ourselves to exceed what we believe are our limitations. And we surprise ourselves when we move to the next level!

If you are more athletic and these workouts are a breeze, then add more repetitions. Adding 10 repetitions to each exercise should definitely give you a challenge. Listen to your body and feel it as you push it. If you can't feel the burn in your muscles, keep going until you do. If you get really sore or are extremely tired, rest for a day and then push it hard the next day after a thorough warm-up.

Goals and Expectations

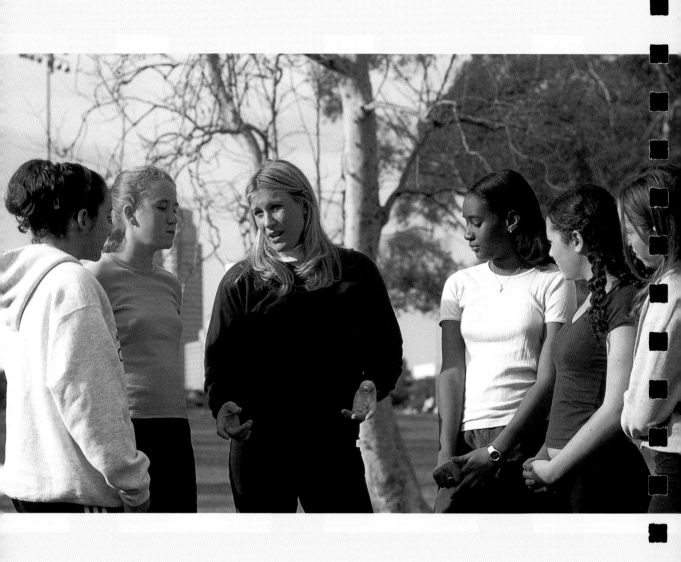

a s a young role model, I think actress Kate Winslet, star of *Titanic*, has one of the best attitudes in Hollywood when it comes to fitness.

"I am who I am," she says. "I'm healthy. I swim a mile every day. I'll never be a stick insect, and I wouldn't want to be either, because it seems to me that a lot of people who are very thin are just really unhappy.

"I had a time in my life when I was about nineteen and I was very thin, and I wasn't eating. I was anorexic for about six months, and I was so unhappy. And someone said to me one day, 'Don't you realize how much of your day you are spending thinking about your physicality?' And it was true. I realized I'd wake up in the morning, the first thing I'd do was look in the mirror: 'Oh, my bum looks big. Oh, my face is fat.' And I just felt, 'What am I doing to my life? I can't even think about others.'

"I feel for those people [anorexics] because they're being screwed up by what is said to be beautiful and successful these days, thin and pretty, and it's just 'a crock.'

"Because of the person I am, I won't be knocked down—ever. They can do what they like," she says. "They can say I'm fat, I'm thin, I'm whatever, and I'll never stop. I just won't. I've got too much to do. I've too much to be happy about."

I'm not proud of things I did to my body before I became a fitness trainer, or after. In retrospect, I feel I was a hypocrite. Here I was teaching others how to live a healthier life with the proper nutrition and exercise, while I was destroying my body—all for the sake of *thin*. But I have come full circle, and now treat my body with the respect it deserves, including giving it nutritious meals, healthy snacks, and plenty of exercise. This lifestyle makes it possible for me to live each day of my life to the fullest. It is a lifestyle I teach my clients and instill into my family—especially my young sons.

Every day I ask my twin boys, Payton and Cooper, to tell me something that they've done that's good for their bodies—whether it's eating a bowl of strawberries or taking a gymnastics class—and we discuss how it's helping them become stronger, healthier boys. And even baby Walker, barely a year old, has started getting fit just by watching the good habits his older brothers are developing. Like most babies, he loves to imitate! What better way to learn?

When I think back on my teenage years, I get a smile on my face. I loved writing this book. Reminiscing on this period of my life brought back many memories that I truly enjoyed.

Being a teen is a great time in your life. You are filled with boundless energy, faced with endless challenges, and learning new things, about yourself and life in general, every day. Remember that the habits and routines you establish now will shape and determine the course of much of your adult life. Use my stories, tips, ideas, workouts, and goals today to help you have the best of all possible tomorrows. Exercise and eating may seem like a small part of your busy life. They really are the most important.

Taking care of your body began the day you were born, as your parents loved and nurtured it. Continue caring for it the same way—don't wait until it's too late. It's the only one you'll ever get and it's the biggest responsibility you'll ever have.

Appendix

There's always more to learn, especially if you want to remain motivated and on top of the fitness world. Here are some of my favorite sources for fitness and health information and support.

Videos for home workouts:

Kathy Kaehler Fitness System—Available at Amazon.com

Cindy Crawford and Kathy Kaehler's "A New Dimension"— Available at Babystyle.com

Target & Tone by Kathy Kaehler—Available at Amazon.com

On the internet:

Sephora.com

gophysical.com

Monthly column:

Self magazine

Recommended apparel:

The Enell Sports Bra (Drew Barrymore's favorite!)
Call (800) 828-7661
Nike shoes and apparel, www.nike.com

Equipment:

Super Rope (The best jump rope of its kind in the world!)
Call (414) 257-3193
Exercise balls, www.relaxtheback.com
Mats, weights, bands, and other exercise equipment
Call (800) 321-6975

For more information on milk and fruit, check out these websites:
For fruit, log on to www.cffa.org
For milk, log on to www.whymilk.com

about the author

Kathy Kaehler, NBC's *Today* show fitness expert has also been the personal trainer to Julia Roberts, Michelle Pfeiffer, Drew Barrymore, Cindy Crawford, Alfre Woodard, Samuel L. Jackson, Penelope Ann Miller, and Claire Forlani, among many others. Kaehler also writes a monthly column for *Self* magazine and is the fitness consultant for Sephora.com. She attended Michigan's Hope College, where she earned a B.S. in physical education with an emphasis in exercise science and dance. On top of everything else, Kaehler is a wife and mother of twin boys and a new baby.

Connie Church, a bestselling writer, has written several books covering a wide range of topics, including fitness, health, beauty, fashion, and psychology. She lives in Los Angeles.

Notes

Notes

Notes

Notes

Notes

Teenage Fitness